全国高等医药院校药学类专业第二轮实验双语教材

药物色谱分析实验与指导

主　　编　郑　枫

副主编　苏梦翔　张珍英

编　　者　(以姓氏笔画为序)

陈　磊（天津大学）

陈金龙（中国药科大学）

张珍英（广东药科大学）

吴春勇（中国药科大学）

苏梦翔（中国药科大学）

郑　枫（中国药科大学）

姜　珍（沈阳药科大学）

闻　俊（海军军医大学）

洪俊丽（南京医科大学）

黄　寅（中国药科大学）

中国健康传媒集团

中国医药科技出版社

内容提要

　　《药物色谱分析实验与指导》是"全国高等医药院校药学类专业第二轮实验双语教材"系列之一，全书采用中英文双语编写，包括药物气相色谱分析、药物高效液相色谱分析、色谱技术在药物鉴定中的应用、色谱技术在体内药物分析中的应用和色谱联用技术在药物分析中的应用等五章内容。本书为书网融合教材，即纸质教材有机融合电子教材、教学配套资源、数字化教学服务（在线教学、在线作业、在线考试），使教学资源更加多样化、立体化。

　　本书适用于药学类本科师生使用，亦可供从事药物色谱分析工作的相关专业人员参考。

图书在版编目（CIP）数据

药物色谱分析实验与指导／郑枫主编. —北京：中国医药科技出版社，2019.12

全国高等医药院校药学类专业第二轮实验双语教材

ISBN 978 - 7 - 5214 - 1338 - 0

Ⅰ.①药… Ⅱ.①郑… Ⅲ.①色谱法 - 应用 - 药物分析 - 实验 - 双语教学 - 医学院校 - 教学参考资料 - 汉、英 Ⅳ.①R917 - 33

中国版本图书馆 CIP 数据核字（2019）第 301304 号

美术编辑 陈君杞
版式设计 南博文化

出版 **中国健康传媒集团** | 中国医药科技出版社
地址 北京市海淀区文慧园北路甲 22 号
邮编 100082
电话 发行：010 - 62227427 邮购：010 - 62236938
网址 www.cmstp.com
规格 889 × 1194mm ¹⁄₁₆
印张 11
字数 244 千字
版次 2019 年 12 月第 1 版
印次 2022 年 9 月第 2 次印刷
印刷 三河市万龙印装有限公司
经销 全国各地新华书店
书号 ISBN 978 - 7 - 5214 - 1338 - 0
定价 **35.00 元**

获取新书信息、投稿、
为图书纠错，请扫码
联系我们。

教学是学校人才培养的中心环节，实验教学是这一环节的重要组成部分。"全国高等医药院校药学类专业实验双语教材"是中国药科大学坚持药学实践教学改革，突出提高学生动手能力、创新思维，通过承担教育部"世行贷款21世纪初高等教育教学改革项目"等多项教改课题，逐步建设完善的一套与药学各专业学科理论课程紧密结合的高水平双语实验教材。

本轮修订，适逢"全国高等医药院校药学类专业第五轮规划教材"及《中国药典》（2020年版）、新版《国家执业药师资格考试大纲》出版，整套教材的修订强调了与新版理论教材知识的结合，与《中国药典》（2020年版）等新颁布的法典法规结合。为更好地服务于新时期高等院校药学教育与人才培养的需要，在上一版的基础上，进一步体现了各门实验课程自身独立性、系统性和科学性，又充分考虑到各门实验课程之间的联系与衔接，主要突出了以下特点。

1. 适应医药行业对人才的要求，体现行业特色，契合新时期药学人才需求的变化，使修订后的教材符合《中国药典》（2020年版）等国家标准及新版《国家执业药师资格考试大纲》等行业最新要求。

2. 更新完善内容，打造教材精品。在上版教材基础上进一步优化、精炼和充实内容。紧密结合"全国高等医药院校药学类专业第五轮规划教材"，强调与实际需求相结合，进一步提高教材质量。

3. 为适应信息化教学的需要，本轮教材全部打造成为书网融合教材，即纸质教材与数字教材、配套教学资源、题库系统、数字化教学服务有机融合，为读者提供全免费增值服务。

4. 坚持双语体系，强调素质培养教材以实践教学为突破口，采用双语体系编写有利于加快药学教育国际接轨，提高学生的科技英语水平，进一步提升学生整体素质。

"全国高等医药院校药学类专业第二轮实验双语教材"历经15年4次建设，在各个时期广大编者的努力下，在广大使用教材师生的支持下日臻完善。本轮教材的出版，必将对推动新时期我国高等药学教育的发展产生积极而深远的影响。希望广大师生在教学实践中对本套教材提出宝贵意见，以便今后进一步修订完善，共同打造精品教材。

吴晓明

全国高等医药院校药学类专业第五轮规划教材常务编委会主任委员

2019年10月

色谱技术是药物分析中必不可少的一种高效分离分析方法,已广泛应用于药物研发、生产流通、乃至临床使用的各个领域;色谱分离技术的应用比例逐渐占据主导地位。我国对药品质量监管要求不断提高,《中国药典》对药物的质量控制方法也在与时俱进。因此,药物色谱分析实验教学已成为药学教育重要的内容之一。

《药物色谱分析实验与指导》以中国药科大学药物分析系开设的药物色谱分析实验课程实践为基础,选取了现行版《中国药典》中收录的薄层色谱法、气相色谱法、高效液相色谱法、色谱联用技术等色谱分析技术,以色谱技术在药物分析中的应用为主线,使学习者能够理论联系实际,掌握常用的色谱分析技术以解决药物分析中的实际问题。从应用对象上,本书主要选取了代表性的化学原料药及其制剂,同时亦兼顾体内药物分析的实验课程需求。

本书采用中英文双语编写,共分为药物气相色谱分析、药物高效液相色谱分析、色谱技术在药物鉴定中的应用、色谱技术在体内药物分析中的应用和色谱联用技术在药物分析中的应用等五章内容。其中药物气相色谱分析包含气相色谱法的基本操作及其在药物含量测定、辅料含量测定、有机溶剂残留测定中的应用,涉及直接进样法、顶空进样法和程序升温法等常用气相色谱技术;药物高效液相色谱分析包含高效液相色谱法的基本操作及其在原料药质量控制、液体制剂质量控制、固体制剂质量控制、有关物质控制中的应用,涉及离子对色谱法、离子抑制色谱法、梯度洗脱法、手性高效液相色谱法等高效液相色谱技术;色谱技术在药物鉴定中的应用包含薄层色谱法、气相色谱法和高效液相色谱法的应用实验;色谱技术在体内药物分析中的应用涉及液液沉淀法、液液萃取法和固相萃取法等前处理技术;色谱联用技术在药物分析中的应用包含气质联用技术和液质联用技术在定性定量分析中的应用。

本书编写分工如下:第一章由广东药科大学张珍英、海军军医大学闻俊编写,第二章由中国药科大学郑枫、沈阳药科大学姜珍、天津大学陈磊编写,第三章由中国药科大学陈金龙、吴春勇编写,第四章由中国药科大学苏梦翔编写,第五章由中国药科大学黄寅、南京医科大学洪俊丽编写,郑枫编写了本教材的大纲并审校全书。感谢中国药科大学药物分析系、中国药科大学教务处和参编院校对本书编写的关心和支持。

本书适用于药学类本科师生使用,亦可供从事药物色谱分析工作的相关专业人员参考。

因编者水平和编写时间所限,书中难免有疏忽错误之处,敬请广大读者批评指正。

编 者

2019 年 10 月

第一章 药物气相色谱分析

Chapter 1 Gas Chromatographic Analysis of Pharmaceuticals

实验一 气相色谱法基本技能实验

【实验目的】

1. 学习气相色谱仪的结构和工作原理。
2. 学习气相色谱法的操作流程。
3. 学习影响气相色谱分离效能的因素。

【实验原理】

1. 气相色谱仪的结构和工作原理 以气体为流动相的色谱法称为气相色谱法（gas chromatography，GC）。气相色谱仪主要包括气路系统、进样系统、分离（柱）系统、检测系统和数据记录处理系统。如图1－1所示，气路系统中的载气由高压钢瓶供给，经减压阀（1）、气体净化器（2）和稳压阀（3）后，以恒定的流速依次流过汽化室（6）、色谱柱和检测器。目前在气相色谱中以毛细管色谱柱为主，由于毛细管色谱柱内径较小，因此载气中大部分气体会通过分流调节阀（8）经分流气路出口（7）排出，进入柱子的流量 F_c 与通过分流阀放空的流量 $F_{分流}$ 之比称为分流比。分流比会严重影响色谱峰形和分离效果，因此分流比的优化是毛细管气相色谱条件优化的重要环节。当载气流出色谱柱进入检测器之前，再通过尾吹气调节阀（9）补足气体流量。

样品由进样系统中的进样器（5）进样，在汽化室（6）高温气化，然后被载气带入分离系统中的色谱柱进行分离。分离系统包括色谱柱和柱温箱（10），色谱柱中的固定相起保留作用，柱温箱控制的柱温对于色谱洗脱和分离具有重要作用。被分离后的样品组分再被载气带入检测器进行响应和检测，并将其转化为电信号，然后传输到放大器，由工作站采集并记录。

2. 色谱分离效能的评价指标 气相色谱和高效液相色谱的分离效能评价指标主要由理论塔板数、分离度、对称因子和重复性等组成。

理论塔板数 n 是在选定的条件下用于评价色谱柱分离待测物的柱效的参数，理论塔板数越高说明色谱柱的分离柱效越高，可以通过改变色谱柱的柱长、内径和固定相提高理论塔板数。毛细管气相色谱的理论塔板数可达 $10^5 \sim 10^6$，分离效能较高，因此可以分离沸点十分相近的组分和极为复杂的多组分混合物。在毛细管气相色谱分析中，分流比对于理论塔板数有重要影响。

扫码"学一学"

扫码"看一看"

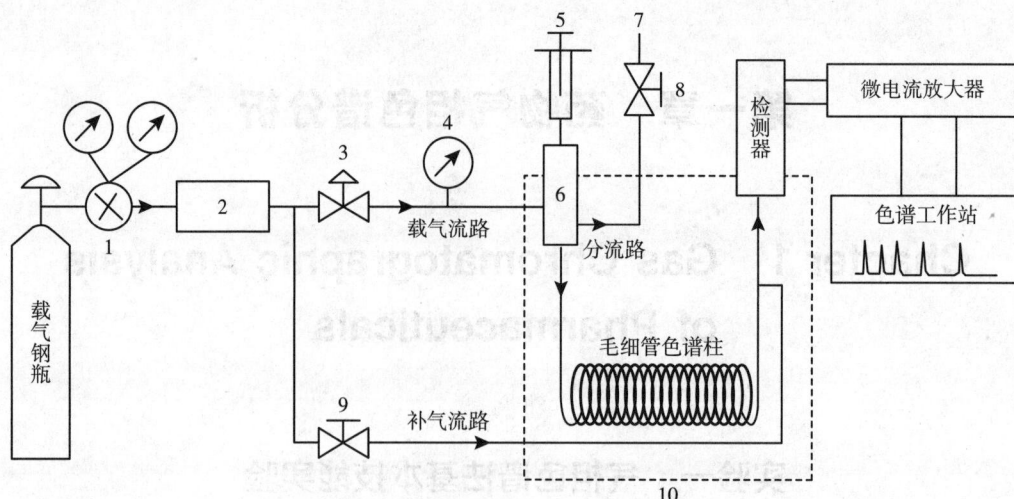

图 1-1　气相色谱仪示意图（毛细管色谱柱）

1. 减压阀；2. 气体净化器；3. 稳压阀；4. 压力表；5. 进样器；6. 汽化室；
7. 分流气路出口；8. 分流调节阀；9. 尾吹气调节阀；10. 柱温箱

分离度 R 是在选定的条件下待测物色谱峰之间的分离效能，R 大于 1.5 时待测物之间达到完全分离，可以通过更换不同色谱柱和改变色谱柱柱温提高分离度。

色谱峰的对称因子（T）反映了待测物色谱峰的对称性，其与柱效和分离度密切相关，主要取决于待测物的性质和所选用的色谱柱，T 在 0.95~1.05 之间时色谱峰呈完全对称。

重复性指连续进样后，色谱峰的保留时间和组分峰面积的相对标准偏差，反映色谱方法的稳定性。气相色谱中由于分流比的因素，导致峰面积的重复性较差，一般需要采用内标法，以组分峰面积与内标峰面积之间的比值进行定量以确保良好的重复性。

【仪器与试剂】

1. 仪器　气相色谱仪，FID 检测器，高纯氮气，氢气，空气，分析天平，微量注射器（100μl），量瓶（10ml、100ml），移液管（1ml、10ml），气相手动进样针（1μl）。

2. 试剂　苯、甲苯为分析纯试剂，甲醇为色谱纯试剂。

【实验内容】

1. 测试溶液的配制　分别配制 50μg/ml 苯的甲醇溶液、50μg/ml 甲苯的甲醇溶液、50μg/ml 苯和甲苯的混合甲醇溶液。

2. 色谱条件的设置　色谱柱：Wondacap-5 毛细管熔融石英毛细管柱（30m×0.32mm×0.25μm）或同类型色谱柱；载气：氮气；柱内流量：4ml/min，分流比 1:20（或根据优化结果选择）；进样口温度：200℃；FID 检测器温度：250℃；柱温 100℃（或根据优化结果选择）；尾吹气为氮气，燃气为氢气，设定流速 30ml/min，助燃气为空气，设定流速 300ml/min。进样量为 1μl。

3. 柱温的优化　选择不同的柱温（80℃、100℃、120℃）考察色谱分离效能。在每次设定的温度下，吸取 1μl 苯的甲醇溶液注入进样口，待组分出峰完毕，停止采集，记录苯的色谱峰保留时间；吸取 1μl 甲苯的甲醇溶液进样，待组分出峰完毕，停止采集，记录色谱峰的保留时间；再吸取 1μl 的苯和甲苯的混合溶液进样，记录苯和甲苯的保留时间、峰面积、理论塔板数、分离度、对称因子，并重复进样 3 次考察重复性。

该项实验主要考察柱温对理论塔板数、分离度、对称因子和重复性的影响，并选择最优柱温。

4. 分流比的优化　选择最优柱温，设定不同分流比（1∶10、1∶20、1∶30）。在每次设定的分流比下，按照柱温优化的实验操作进行分流比的考察。该项实验主要考察不同分流比对理论塔板数、分离度、对称因子和重复性的影响，并选择最优的进样分流比。

【数据记录与处理】

1. 柱温优化数据记录

表 1-1　柱温优化的数据记录

柱温 (℃)	序号	色谱峰 (苯) t_R (min)	色谱峰 (甲苯) t_R (min)	苯和甲苯混合液 色谱峰 (苯) t_R (min)	A_1	n	T	色谱峰 (甲苯) t_R (min)	A_2	n	T	R	色谱峰 (苯和甲苯) A_1/A_2
80	1												
	2												
	3												
100	1												
	2												
	3												
120	1												
	2												
	3												

注：表中 t_R 为保留时间，A 为峰面积，n 为理论塔板数，T 为对称因子，R 为分离度。

2. 分流比优化数据记录

表 1-2　分流比优化的数据记录

分流比	序号	色谱峰 (苯) t_R (min)	色谱峰 (甲苯) t_R (min)	苯和甲苯混合液 色谱峰 (苯) t_R (min)	A_1	n	T	色谱峰 (甲苯) t_R (min)	A_2	n	T	R	色谱峰 (苯和甲苯) A_1/A_2
1∶10	1												
	2												
	3												

分流比	序号	色谱峰（苯）	色谱峰（甲苯）	苯和甲苯混合液									
				色谱峰（苯）				色谱峰（甲苯）				色谱峰（苯和甲苯）	
		t_R (min)	t_R (min)	t_R (min)	A_1	n	T	t_R (min)	A_2	n	T	R	A_1/A_2
1:20	1												
	2												
	3												
1:30	1												
	2												
	3												

注：表中 t_R 为保留时间，A 为峰面积，n 为理论塔板数，T 为对称因子，R 为分离度。

3. 柱温优化结果

表 1-3　柱温优化结果

柱温（℃）		苯和甲苯混合液							
		苯			甲苯			苯和甲苯	
		A_1	n	T	A_2	n	T	R	A_1/A_2
80	平均值								
	$RSD\%$								
100	平均值								
	$RSD\%$								
120	平均值								
	$RSD\%$								

注：表中 $RSD\%$ 为相对标准偏差，A 为峰面积，n 为理论塔板数，T 为对称因子，R 为分离度。

4. 分流比优化结果

表 1-4　分流比优化结果

分流比		苯和甲苯混合液							
		苯			甲苯			苯和甲苯	
		A_1	n	T	A_2	n	T	R	A_1/A_2
1:10	平均值								
	$RSD\%$								
1:20	平均值								
	$RSD\%$								
1:30	平均值								
	$RSD\%$								

注：表中 $RSD\%$ 为相对标准偏差，A 为峰面积，n 为理论塔板数，T 为对称因子，R 为分离度。

【讨论与指导】

1. 气相色谱仪的基本操作方法

（1）开机　仪器操作前检查载气气压是否足够，气路是否完整连接，并将色谱柱接至进样口和检测器的相应接口上。确定无误后，打开载气气源阀门，调节表头上的减压阀，使载气流速控制在所需要的流速值（气压一般在 0.3～0.6MPa）；依次打开 GC 主机、氢气发生器、空气发生器、控制电脑的电源。

（2）设置参数　打开色谱工作站，连接仪器，进入 GC 实时分析窗口；在参数设置目录下，逐项完成数据采集设置（检测器、采样速率、结束时间），温度设置（进样口、柱温箱和检测器），进样口设置（进样模式、压力、总流量、吹扫流量、色谱柱流、气流线速度、分流比），检测器设置（尾吹流量、氢气流量、空气流量）。若进行程序升温，同时还应设置升温程序（按程序逐项设置温度、速率、保留时间）。设置完毕点击"下载"或"确定"。

若已经保存过色谱分析方法，只需调入方法文件（如：点击"文件"→点击"方法文件"→选择路径→选择文件）进行实验。

（3）进样与数据采集　检查设定的各项参数无误后，开始运行仪器（如点击"开启GC"），检测器、进样器和色谱柱开始升温；待各项参数均达到预设值时，在工作站下点击查看色谱基线，观察色谱基线是否平稳；待色谱基线稳定后，先进行样品信息的录入，再用进样针量取指定体积的试样，注射到进样口，立即点击"开始"按钮，即开始采样。观察出峰情况，直到所有组分出峰完毕，停止采集，保存色谱图文件。在离线工作站打开文件，调出所保存的色谱图和数据，进行数据处理。

（4）关机　样品测定完毕后，对柱温、进样器温度、检测器温度进行降温设置（设置温度一定要低于100℃）；当柱温、进样器温度、检测器温度达到设定值，依次关闭氢气发生器、空气压缩机、控制电脑、气相色谱仪主机电源，最后关闭载气。如有必要卸下色谱柱，并及时按色谱柱说明书对色谱柱进行保养。

2. 气相色谱使用的注意事项

（1）色谱柱安装时，毛细管色谱柱两端切口要平齐，长时间不用或新的柱子要两端各切掉 2cm 左右。

（2）开机前检查气路系统是否有漏气。硅橡胶垫在几十次进样后，容易漏气，需及时更换。

（3）进样前，必须按先通载气，再开电源，最后升温的顺序操作；试验结束后，按先降温、再关电源，最后关载气的顺序操作。

（4）用微量注射器取液体试样，应先用少量试样洗涤多次，再慢慢抽入试样，并稍多于需要量。如内有气泡则将针头朝上，使气泡上升排出，再将过量的试样排出，用滤纸吸去针尖外所沾试样。注意切勿使针头内的试样流失。进样量不宜过大，填充柱一般不大于 2μl，毛细管柱进样量不宜大于 1μl。

（5）样品进针要迅速，如果针在汽化室内滞留时间过长，针头部分的溶液也汽化，容易造成定量不准。

（6）保持每次进样的平行性，这将直接影响测定结果的重现性。

（7）温度设置时，一定不能超过仪器部件的最高使用温度，最高升温速率。通常柱温比固定液最高温度低30℃，检测器温度至少比柱温高30℃，汽化室温度通常与检测器温度相近。

（8）进样分析前，一定要检查各项参数是否已达设定值，FID 检测器是否点着火。确保仪器已达设定条件，并 FID 已点着火的情况下，开始进样分析。

（9）设定方法条件参数后，一定要按"下载"或"确定"，此时所设定条件方可执行运行。

（10）关闭仪器时，一定要降温至设定值时，才能关闭仪器。

Experiment 1 Basic Skill Experiment of Gas Chromatography

1. Experimental purposes

1.1 To learn the structure and working principle of GC instrument.

1.2 To learn the operating procedures of GC method.

1.3 To learn factors affecting the separation efficiency of GC.

2. Experimental principles

2.1 The structure and working principle of gas chromatographic instrument

Gas chromatography (GC) is a kind of chromatographic method with chemically inert gas as the mobile phase. A gas chromatographic instrument is mainly made up of carrier gas system, sample injection system, separation (column) system, detection system and data recording and processing system. As shown in Fig. 1 – 1, the carrier gas throughout the chromatograph is supplied by a high pressureized cylinder, which is followed by passing through the press regulator (1), the gas purifier (2) and the pressure stabilizing valve (3) to obtain a constant gas press. After a two – stage pressure regulator, the carrier gas flows into the vaporization chamber (6) and the chromatographic column, and finally reaches the detector successively at constant flow rate. At present, capillary columns are widely used in gas chromatography for both the fast separation speed and the high number of theoretical plates. But most of carrier gas will be discharged by sample splitters including split gas outlet (7) of split valve (8) because of the lower capacity of capillary columns. The ratio of the flow F_c into the column to the flow F through the split gas outlet is called the split ratio. It will seriously affect the chromatographic peak shape and resolution, so the optimization of split ratio is an important step in capillary gas chromatography conditions setting. Before the carrier gas out of the column enters the detector, the gas flow is supplemented by the tail blowing regulating valve (9).

Samples are rapidly injected by means of a microsyringe (5) through a silicone rubber septum into vaporization chamber (6) in sample injection port where the sample is vaporized at high temperature. Then the vaporized samples are carried by carrier gas into the chromatographic colum being hosed in the column oven (10) for separation. Thus the separation system normally includes the chromatographic column and the column oven. The stationary phase in the chromatographic column plays a retention role, and the column temperature controlled by the column oven is an important variable in the chromatographic elution and separation. The separated components are automatically detected by the detector as they emerge from the column and their responses are converted into electrical signals, which are transmitted to the amplifier for collection and record by the workstation.

2.2 The evaluation indexes for chromatographic separation efficiency

The number of theoretical plates, the resolution and the symmetry factor are important indexes for the chromatographic separation. The reproducibility is also important for the chromatographic methods.

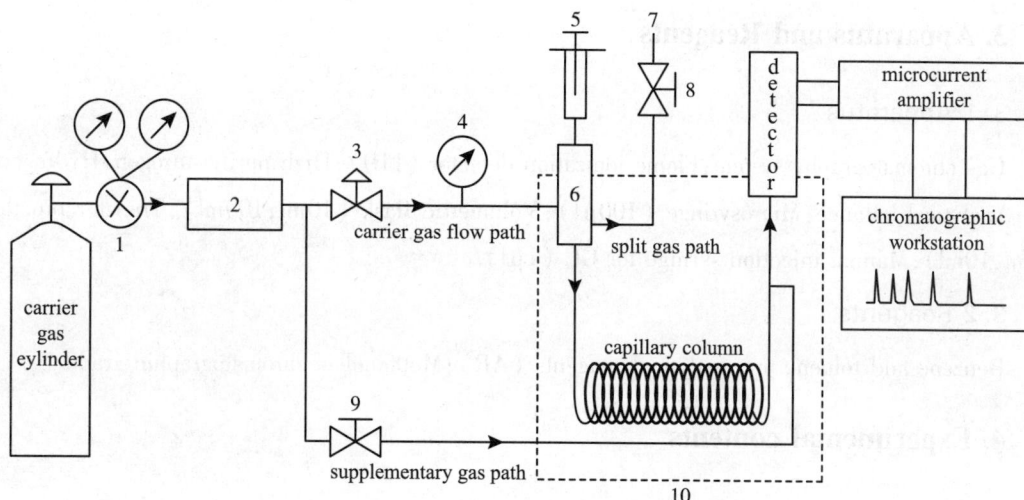

Fig. 1 – 1   The schematic diagram of a chromatographic instrument (capillary column).

1. Pressure regulator; 2. Gas purifier; 3. Pressure stabilizing valve; 4. Pressure gauge; 5. Microsyringe; 6. Vaporization chamber;

7. Split gas outlet; 8. Split valve; 9. Tail blowing regulating valve; 10. Column oven

The number of theoretical plates (n) is a parameter used to evaluate the chromatographic column efficiency under the selected conditions. The higher number of theoretical plates means the higher separation efficiency of the chromatographic column. The number of theoretical plates can be increased by lengthening the column, decreasing the inner diameter of column and optimizing the composition of the stationary phase. Capillary gas chromatography provides extremely high separation efficiency by the number of theoretical plates reaching $10^5 - 10^6$. Therefore, the components with very similar boiling point and very complex multi – component mixtures can be separated by capillary GC. In capillary gas chromatography, adjustment of the split ratio is also a convenient method to improving the number of theoretical plates.

The resolution (R) represents the separation efficiency between chromatographic peaks under the selected conditions. When R is greater than 1. 5, it means the efficient separation with baseline resolution. Separation can be improved by replacing different chromatographic columns and decreasing column temperature.

The symmetry factor (T) of peaks reflects the symmetry of the chromatographic peak, which is closely related to the column efficiency and separation. It mainly depends on the properties of the measured components and the selected chromatographic column. When T is between 0. 95 and 1. 05, the chromatographic peak is completely symmetrical.

Reproducibility refers to the relative standard deviations of the retention time and the peak, which is area after continuous injection, which reflects the stability of chromatographic methods. The split ratio is one of the factors crucially decreases the reproducibility of the separational performance of capillary columns. The internal standard method is usually used to improve the reproducibility. Good reproducibility can be obtained by measuring the ratio between the peak areas of the measured components and the internal standard.

3. Apparatus and Reagents

3.1 Apparatus

Gas chromatography system; Flame ionization detector (FID); High purity nitrogen; Hydrogen; Air; Analytical balance; Microsyringe (100μl); Volumetric flask (10ml, 100ml); Transfer pipettes (1ml, 10ml); Manual injection syringe for GC (1μl).

3.2 Reagents

Benzene and toluene are analytical reagents (AR); Methanol is chromatographic grade.

4. Experimental contents

4.1 Preparation of test solutions

Methanol solution of 50μg/ml benzene, methanol solution of 50μg/ml toluene, and the mixed methanol solution of 50μg/ml benzene and 50μg/ml toluene are prepared respectively.

4.2 Setting of gas chromatography conditions

Wondacap-5 fused silica capillary column (30m×0.32mm×0.25μm) or similar columns is used as the stationary phase.

The carrier gas is nitrogen. The column flow is about 4ml/min and the split ratio is 1 : 20 or according to the optimization results.

The inlet temperature and hydrogen flame detector temperature are 200℃ and 250℃, respectively.

The column temperature is 100℃ or according to the optimization results. The tail blowing gas is nitrogen.

The 30ml/min of hydrogen is used as the burning gas. Air as assistant gas is set at 300ml/min.

The inject volume is 1μl.

4.3 Optimization of column temperature conditions

The column temperature is optimized at three different values of 80℃, 100℃ and 120℃.

Under the chromatographic conditions above set, for each column temperature, inject 1μl of the methanol solution of benzene into the gas chromatography system, stop acquirement and record the retention time of benzene following complete elution of all components; inject 1μl of the methanol solution of toluene into the gas chromatography system, after complete elution of all components, stop acquirement and record the retention time of toluene. Then inject 1μl of the mixed solution of benzene and toluene and record their retention times, peak areas, the number of theoretical plates, symmetry factors, the resolution, and the reproducibility by repeating injection three times.

These experiments mainly are used to investigate the influence of column temperature on the number of theoretical plates, resolution, symmetry factors and reproducibilities. And then the optimal column temperature will be selected according to the above experimental results.

4. 4 Optimization of the split ratio

At the optimal column temperature, different split ratios of 1 : 10,1 : 20 and 1 : 30 are set for the optimization.

For each split ratio, the experimental procedures are the same as those in optimization of column temperature conditions.

These experiments mainly are used to investigate the influence of split ratio on the number of theoretical plates, resolution, symmetry factors and reproducibility, and then select the optimal split ratio.

5. Data record and processing

5. 1 The records for the optimization of column temperature

Table 1 –1　The record for the optimization of column temperature

Column temperature (℃)		Benzene t_R	Toluene t_R	The mixed solution of benzene and toluene									
				Benzene				Toluene					
				t_R	A_1	n	T	t_R	A_2	n	T	R	A_1/A_2
80	1												
	2												
	3												
100	1												
	2												
	3												
120	1												
	2												
	3												

Note: t_R is retention time; A is peak area; n is the number of theoretical plates; T is symmetric factor; R is resolution.

5. 2 The records for the optimization of split ratio

Table 1 –2　The record for the optimization of split ratio

Split ratio		Benzene t_R	Toluene t_R	The mixed solution of benzene and toluene									
				Benzene				Toluene					
				t_R	A_1	n	T	t_R	A_2	n	T	R	A_1/A_2
1 : 10	1												
	2												
	3												
1 : 20	1												
	2												
	3												
1 : 30	1												
	2												
	3												

Note: t_R is retention time; A is peak area; n is the number of theoretical plates; T is symmetric factor; R is resolution.

5. 3 The results for the optimization of column temperature

Table 1 – 3   The results for the optimization of column temperature

Column temperature (°C)		The mixed solution of benzene and toluene							
		Benzene			Toluene				
		A_1	n	T	A_2	n	T	R	A_1/A_2
80	AVE								
	RSD%								
100	AVE								
	RSD%								
120	AVE								
	RSD%								

Note: *RSD%* is the relative standard deviation; *A* is peak area; *n* is the number of theoretical plates; *T* is the symmetric factor; *R* is resolution.

5. 4 The results forthe optimization of split ratio

Table 1 – 4   The results for the optimization of split ratio

Split ratio		The mixed solution of benzene and toluene							
		Benzene			Toluene				
		A_1	n	T	A_2	n	T	R	A_1/A_2
1 : 10	AVE								
	RSD%								
1 : 20	AVE								
	RSD%								
1 : 30	AVE								
	RSD%								

Note: *RSD%* is the relative standard deviation; *A* is peak area; *n* is the number of theoretical plates; *T* is the symmetric factor; *R* is resolution.

6. Discussion and guidance

6. 1 Basic operation of GC

a. Starting up   Before the operation of the instrument, check whether the carrier gas pressure is sufficient and the gas path is completely connected. Then connect the chromatographic column to the corresponding interface of the injection port and detector. After confirmation, open the carrier gas source valve and adjust the pressure regulator on the gauge head, so that the carrier gas flow can be controlled at the required flow (gas pressure is generally 0. 3 ~ 0. 6 Mpa). Turn on the powers of GC controller, hydrogen generator, air compressor and PC.

b. Setting parameters   Start the chromatographic workstation to connect the instruments and enter the GC real – time analysis window. Under the parameter setting catalogue, complete data acquisition settings (detector, sampling rate, end time), temperature settings (injection port temperature, column temperature, detector temperature), injection settings (injection model, pressure, total flow, purge flow, column flow, gas linear velocity, split ratio), detector settings (tail blowing flow, hydrogen flow, air flow). If the temperature programming technique is applied, the program should also be set up (temperature, heating rate and holding time shall be set item by item according to the program). After setting up, click "download" or "ok".

If the chromatographic analysis method has been saved, simply load the method file (for example: click "file" → click "method file" → select file path → select file) to carry out the experiment.

c. Injection and data acquisition　After confirmation of all parameters set correctly, start running the instrument (for example, click "start GC"). Then the detector, injection port and chromatographic column start heating up. When all the parameters reach the preset values, click the "monitor baseline" to ensure that the baseline of the detector is stable. After the creation of sample information in the workstation, take a specified volume of sample with the injection microsyringe and inject it quickly it into the injection port. Click the "start" button immediately to start sampling and observe the chromatogram until all components are eluted completely. Then stop the acquisition and save all data.

Open the chromatogram in the offline workstation for the data processing.

d. Turning off　After the analysis of sample, start the cooling of column, injection port and detector (the temperature must be set lower than 100℃). After the temperatures of column, injector and detector reach the preset value, turn off the powers of hydrogen generator, air compressor, PC, gas chromatography controller, and finally turn off carrier gas. If necessary, remove and maintain the column in time according to the column specifications.

6. 2 Notes for the use of GC

a. Before the chromatographic column is installed, the two ends of the column should be cut off about 2cm each for a new column or a column without being used for a long time, and then the incisions at both ends of the capillary column should be smoothed.

b. Check the gas circuit system throughout chromatograph for gas leakage before the operation. A silicone rubber septum is often destroyed to leak after dozens of injections and needs to be replaced in time.

c. Before injecting samples, it must be operated in the order of loading gas first, then turning on the power, and finally heating up. After analysis completion, it should follow the order: first cooling down, then turning off the power, and finally closing the carrier gas.

d. When taking liquid samples with a microsyringe, the microsyringe should be washed several times by a small amount of samples, then slowly take the samples slightly more than the required amount. If there are bubbles in the microsyringe, put the microsyringe upward to rise and remove the bubbles. Then discharge the excess samples and use filter papers to absorb the waste samples outside the tip. Be careful not to lose the sample inside the microsyringe. The amount of samples injected is should be with a suitable size. For ordinary packed analytical columns, the sample amount should be less than $5\mu l$, and capillary columns require samples no more than $1\mu l$.

e. Injection should be finished quickly. If the microsyringe stays in the evaporation chamber for a long time, the solution of the head of injector will be evaporated, which will easily cause an inaccurate quantification.

f. Maintaining each injection at the same matters, the variation of injection will directly affect the reproducibility of the results.

g. When setting the temperature, it must not exceed the maximum operating temperatu – re and the maximum heating rate of the instrument. In general, the column temperature is 30℃ lower than the maximum temperature of the stationary phase, the detector temperature is at least 30℃ higher than the column temperature, and the vaporization chamber temperature is usually close to the detector temperature.

h. Before analysis, it is necessary to ensure that the parameters have reached the set value and the FID detector is on fire.

i. After setting method conditions, do not forget to press "download" or "confirm" to run.

j. When turning off the instrument, the temperature must be below 100℃ before closing the instrument.

扫码"学一学"

实验二 气相色谱法测定风油精中薄荷脑的含量

【实验目的】

1. 学习气相色谱条件的建立与优化过程。
2. 学习气相色谱法测定药物含量的流程。
3. 学习内标法测定药物含量的原理。

【实验原理】

1. 薄荷脑的性状 薄荷脑（图2-1）是风油精中主要成分，其纯品是无色针状结晶体，密度0.89g/cm³，熔点32～36℃，沸点216℃，折射率1.46。它的分子结构是一种饱和的环状醇，具有3个不对称碳原子，而且都存在着旋光异构体，因此总共有12种异构体。本品微溶于水；溶于乙醇、三氯甲烷、乙醚、石油醚、冰醋酸、液体矿脂。薄荷脑生产主要以薄荷油为原料，先将其冷冻析出薄荷脑结晶，然后用离心机分离，最后用升华法或蒸馏法精制而得。

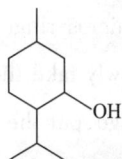

图2-1 薄荷脑的结构

2. 内标法的原理 取对照品溶液和内标溶液混合，配成校正因子测定用的对照溶液。取一定量注入仪器，记录色谱图。测量对照品和内标物质的峰面积或峰高，计算校正因子：

$$校正因子（f）= (A_S / C_S) / (A_R / C_R)$$

式中，A_S 为内标物质的峰面积或峰高；A_R 为对照品的峰面积或峰高；C_S 为内标物质的浓度；C_R 为对照品的浓度。

再取含有内标物质的供试品溶液，注入仪器，记录色谱图，测量供试品中待测成分（或其杂质）和内标物质的峰面积或峰高，按下式计算含量：

$$含量\ (C_X) = f \cdot A_X / (A_S' / C_S')$$

式中，A_X 为供试品的峰面积或峰高；C_X 为供试品的浓度；A_S' 为内标物质的峰面积或峰高；C_S' 为内标物质的浓度；f 为内标法校正因子。

内标法测定结果不受进样量和操作条件变化的影响，因此采用内标法可避免因样品前处理及进样体积误差对结果的影响，在气相色谱中应用较多。

【仪器与试剂】

1. 仪器 气相色谱仪，FID 检测器，高纯氮气，氢气，空气，分析天平，微量注射器（100μl），量瓶（10ml、100ml）、移液管（1ml），气相手动进样针（1μl）。

2. 试剂 风油精（市售品，含薄荷脑 32%）；薄荷脑对照品（中国食品药品检定研究院）；正辛醇（密度为 0.83g/cm³）、乙酸乙酯均为分析纯。

【实验内容】

1. 对照品溶液的配制 取薄荷脑对照品约 100mg，精密称定，置 10ml 量瓶中，精密加入内标正辛醇 100μl，加乙酸乙酯溶解并稀释至刻度，摇匀，作为对照品溶液。

2. 供试品溶液的配制 精密量取风油精 1ml，置 100ml 量瓶中，精密加入内标正辛醇 100μl，加乙酸乙酯溶解并稀释至刻度，摇匀，作为供试品溶液。

3. 色谱条件的设置 色谱柱：Alltech ECONO EC－1 熔融石英毛细管柱（30m × 0.32mm × 1.0μm）或同类型色谱柱；载气：氮气；柱内流量：4ml/min；分流比 1：20；进样口温度：200℃；检测器温度：250℃；FID 检测条件：燃气为氢气，设定流速 30ml/min，助燃气为空气，设定流速 300ml/min。

柱温根据优化结果选择。

4. 柱温的优化 在 90～130℃范围内选择设定不同的柱温，每次取 1μl 对照品溶液注入气相色谱仪，记录乙酸乙酯、正辛醇、薄荷脑的依序出峰时间；取 1μl 供试品溶液注入气相色谱仪，记录薄荷脑与相邻干扰色谱峰的分离度，选择分离度不小于 1.2 的柱温条件用于含量测定。

5. 含量测定 选择合适的柱温条件，精密量取 1μl 对照品溶液注入气相色谱仪，测量至少三次，计算校正因子的平均值；精密量取 1μl 供试品溶液注入气相色谱仪，测定，按内标法测定风油精中薄荷脑的标示量百分含量，取三次测定结果的平均值。

【数据记录与处理】

1. 对照品溶液的配制记录

表 2－1 对照品溶液的配制记录

对照品的称样量	对照品溶液浓度（C_R，g/ml）	内标的计算量	内标物质的浓度（C_S，g/ml）

2. 柱温条件的优化结果

表 2-2 柱温条件的优化结果

柱温	对照品溶液各成分保留时间（min）			样品溶液
	乙酸乙酯	正辛醇	薄荷脑	分离度
90℃				
100℃				
110℃				
120℃				
130℃				

3. 含量测定的原始数据

表 2-3 含量测定的原始数据

	序号	薄荷脑峰面积	正辛醇峰面积
对照品溶液	1		
	2		
	3		
供试品溶液	1		
	2		
	3		

4. 校正因子的计算结果

根据校正因子计算公式：$f = (A_S / C_S) / (A_R / C_R)$，计算每次对照品溶液进样分析所得的校正因子 f，并计算三次进样得到的校正因子平均值 $f_{均}$。

表 2-4 校正因子的计算结果

	第一次	第二次	第三次	平均值
校正因子（f）				

5. 标示量百分含量的计算结果 根据含量计算公式计算供试品溶液中的薄荷脑浓度 $C_X = f_{均} \times A_X / (A_S' / C_S')$，再计算标示量的百分含量 $= (C_X \times D) / S \times 100\%$。$D$ 为风油精样品测定过程中的稀释倍数；S 为风油精中薄荷脑含量的标示量（g/ml）。

表 2-5 标示量百分含量的计算结果

	薄荷脑浓度 C_X	标示量百分含量（%）	稀释倍数 D	标示量 S
第一次				
第二次				
第三次				
平均值				

【讨论与指导】

1. 适合气相色谱分析的样品 在选择使用气相色谱法分析样品时，首先要了解待测物的性质，才能判断其是否可以进行气相色谱分析。气相色谱使用气体为流动相，待测物必须要有一定的蒸气压，在汽化室高温气化后才能被载气带入色谱柱进行分离分析。同时由于需要在高温下进行分析，所以待分析样品同时需要具备热稳定性，不会在气相分析时分解。气相色谱能直接分析的样品通常是气体或液体，固体样品在分析前应当溶解在适当的溶剂中，而且还要保证样品中不含高沸点的组分，否则会污染进样口和色谱柱。因此在对样品进行分析前，需要预先估计其中待测成分的沸点。如果样品较为简单，具有挥发性成分则可以直接分析。如果样品不能直接分析，或者其中待测成分浓度太低，就必须进行必要的预处理，如采用萃取、稀释、提纯、衍生化等方法处理样品，再进行气相色谱分析。

2. 确定气相色谱仪器的配置 气相色谱仪器的配置主要应根据待测样品选择合适的分离与检测条件的选择，如载气、色谱柱、检测器等。

一般应首先确定检测器类型。碳氢化合物常选择 FID 检测器，含电负性基团（F、Cl等）较多且碳氢含量较少的物质易选择 ECD 检测器；对检测灵敏度要求不高，或含有非碳氢化合物组分时，可选择 TCD 检测器；对于含硫、磷的样品可选择 FPD 检测器。

根据待测组分性质选择适合的色谱柱，一般遵循相似相溶规律。分离非极性物质时选择非极性色谱柱，分离极性物质时选择极性色谱柱。色谱柱确定后，根据样本中待测组分分配系数的差值情况，确定色谱柱工作温度，简单体系采用等温方式，分配系数相差较大的复杂体系采用程序升温方式进行分析。

常用的载气包括有氢气、氦气和氮气。由于氢气和氦气的分子量低，常用于填充柱色谱的载气；氮气则常用于毛细管柱色谱的载气。气相色谱 – 质谱联用则以氦气作为载气。

3. 气相色谱条件的优化 当气相色谱仪器的条件准备好之后，就可开始进行尝试性分离。这时要确定初始分离条件，主要包括进样量、进样口温度、检测器温度、色谱柱温度和载气流速。

进样量要根据样品浓度、色谱柱容量和检测器灵敏度来确定。样品浓度不超过 10mg/ml 时填充柱的进样量通常为 1～5μl，而对于毛细管柱，进样量一般不超过 2μl。

进样口温度主要由样品的沸点范围决定，还要考虑色谱柱的使用温度。原则上讲，进样口温度高一些有利，一般要接近样品中沸点最高的组分的沸点，但要低于组分分解温度。检测器的温度一般要略高于进样口温度，不能低于色谱柱温度。

色谱柱柱温是气相色谱中影响色谱分离的主要因素，应根据待测物性质的不同和分离目的的差异，选择合适的柱温条件；每一种色谱柱都有最高使用温度，柱温设置不得高于该最高使用温度。

载气流速主要根据色谱柱的类型确定。对于毛细管柱需要采用分流装置，柱内流量较小（不超过 6ml/min），对于填充柱则可采用更高载气流速。

4. 气相色谱的含量测定方法 常用的气相色谱定量方法有面积归一化法、内标法、外标法和标准溶液加入法。面积归一化法较为简单，仅当样品由同系物组成或者只是为了粗略估算时，才选择该法。外标法是通过供试品和已知浓度对照品中待测物的峰面积进行定量。内标法则以待测物相对于内标物的响应值进行定量，内标物分别加到标准样品和未知样品中，这样就可抵消由于操作条件（包括进样量）的波动带来的误差。标准加入法，是在供试品中定量加入待测物的对照品，然后根据峰面积的增加量来进行定量计算，这是气相色谱中较为特殊的一种定量方法，多用于顶空进样中消除基质效应的影响。

Experiment 2　Determination of Menthol in Fengyoujing by Gas Chromatography

1. Experimental purposes

1. 1 To learn the development and optimization of gas chromatography conditions.

1. 2 To learn the procedures of gas chromatography for the assay.

1. 3 To learn the principle for the assay by the internal standard method.

2. Experimental principles

2. 1 The characters of menthol

Menthol (Fig. 2 – 1) is one of the main ingredients in Fengyoujing. The standard of menthol is a colorless acicular crystal with the density of 0. 89g/cm^3, melting point of 32 ~ 36℃, boiling point of 216℃ and refractive index of 1. 46. There are three asymmetric carbon atoms in the structure of menthol, generating 12 optical isomers. It is slightly soluble in water and freely soluble in dehydrated ethanol, chloroform, ether, petroleum ether, glacial acetic acid and liquid petrolatum. The peppermint oil is the raw material for the production of menthol. Menthol crystals could be derived by the process of freezing peppermint oil firstly, then separated by a centrifugal machine, and finally purified by sublimation or distillation.

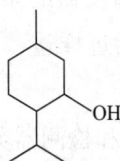

Fig. 2 – 1　The structure of menthol

2. 2 The principle of the internal standard method

The reference solution is prepared by mixing the reference substance solution and the internal standard solution for the determination of the correction factor. Then it is injected into the chromatography system for measuring the peak area or peak height of the reference substance and the internal standard. The correction factor was calculated as follows:

$$\text{Correction factor}(f) = (A_S / C_S) / (A_R / C_R)$$

Where, A_S is the peak area or peak height of the internal standard; A_R is the peak area or peak height of the reference substance; C_S is the concentration of the internal standard; C_R is the concentration of the reference standard.

Then the sample solution containing the internal standard substance is prepared and injected into the chromatography system. The peak area or peak height of the analyte and the internal standard is measured to calculate the content as follows:

$$\text{Content}(C_X) = f \cdot A_X / (A_S' / C_S')$$

Where: A_X is the peak area or peak height of analyte; C_X is the concentration of the sample solution; A_s' is the peak area or the peak height of the internal standard; C_s' is the concentration of the internal standard solution; f is the correction factor in the internal standard method.

The results of the internal standard method are less affected by changes of injection volume and operation conditions. Thus, the internal standard method is often selected in the gas chromatography for the assay.

3. Apparatus and Reagents

3. 1 Apparatus

Gas chromatography system; Flame ionization detector (FID); High purity nitrogen; Hydrogen; Air; Analytical balance; Microsyringe (100μl); Volumetric flask (10ml); Transfer pipettes (1ml); Manual injection syringe for GC (1μl).

3. 2 Reagents

Fengyoujing (commercial products, containing menthol 32%); Menthol reference substance (National institute for the control of pharmaceutical and biological products); n – octanol (density: 0. 83g/cm^3) and ethyl acetate are all analytical reagent (AR).

4. Experimental contents

4. 1 Preparation of the reference solution

Accurately weigh 100mg of menthol reference substance and pipette 100μl of n – octanol to a 10ml volumetric flask, then dissolve them with ethyl acetate to the mark and shake well as the reference solution.

4. 2 Preparation of the sample solution

Accurately pipette 1ml of the sample and 100μl of n – octanol to a 100ml volumetric flask, then dissolve them with ethyl acetate to the mark and shake well as the sample solution.

4. 3 Setting of gas chromatography conditions

Alltech ECONO EC – 1 fused silica capillary column (30m × 0. 32mm × 1. 0μm) or similar columns is used as the stationary phase. The carrier gas is nitrogen. The column flow is about 4ml/min and the split ratio is 1:20. The inlet temperature and hydrogen flame detector temperature are 200℃ and 250℃, respectively. The column temperature is set according to the optimization results.

4. 4 Optimization ofcolumn temperature conditions

The column temperature is optimized at the different value in the range from 90℃ to 130℃. For each run, inject 1μl of the reference solution into the gas chromatography system, and record the retention time of ethyl acetate, n – octanol and menthol; inject 1μl of the sample solution into the gas chromatography system, and record the resolution between the chromatographic peak of menthol and the adjacent peaks. The resolution should be no less than 1. 2 for the assay.

4. 5 Assay

At the optimized temperature, inject 1μl of the reference solution into the gas chromatography system to calculate the correction factor and repeat three times to obtain the average value. Then inject 1μl of the sample solution into the gas chromatography system for the assay by the internal standard method and calculate the percentage of labelled amount of menthol in Fengyoujing according to the results of three times.

5. Data record and processing

5. 1 Record for the preparation of the reference solution

Table 2 – 1　Record for the preparation of the reference solution

Amount of reference substance	Concentration of the reference substance (C_R ,g/ml)	Amount of the internal standard	Concentration of the internal standard (C_S ,g/ml)

5. 2 Optimization ofcolumn temperature conditions

Table 2 – 2　The results of the optimization of column temperature conditions

| Column temperature | Retention time (min) of analytes in the reference solution | | | Sample solution |
	Ethyl acetate	n – octanol	Menthol	Resolution
90℃				
100℃				
110℃				
120℃				
130℃				

5. 3 Original data for assay

Table 2 – 3　The original data for assay

	Number	The peak area of menthol	The peak area of n – octanol
Reference solution	1		
	2		
	3		
Sample solution	1		
	2		
	3		

5. 4 Calculation of the correction factor

Calculate the correction factor according to the following equation：

$$f = (A_S/ C_S)/ (A_R/ C_R)$$

and repeat three times to obtain the average value f_{ave}.

Table 2 – 4　The correction factor results

	1	2	3	f_{ave}
The correction factor(f)				

5. 5 Calculation of the percentage of labelled amount

Calculate the concentration of menthol in the sample solution according to the following equation:

$$C_X = f_{ave} \times A_X / (A_S / C_S)$$

Then the percentage of labelled amount of menthol in Fengyoujing is calculated according to the following equation:

Percentage of the labelled amount $= (C_X \times D)/S \times 100\%$

Where: D is the dilute multiple during the preparation of the sample solution; S is the labelled amount (mg/ml).

Table 2 – 5 The result of the percentage of labelled amount

	Concentration of menthol (C_X)	Percentage of labelled amount(%)	Dilution multiple (D)	Labelled amount (S)
1				
2				
3				
AVE				

6. Discussion and guidance

6. 1 The suitable sample for the GC analysis

The characters of the analytes contribute to the selection of chromatographic method for the analysis. Gas is the mobile phase in the gas chromatography, so only the volatile components can be separated and analyzed in the gas chromatography. Meanwhile, the analytes for GC analysis should be stable under high temperature without being decomposed. Generally, the sample of gas or liquid can be directly analyzed by gas system. Solid sample should be dissolved in a suitable solvent before analysis and the sample must be free of some high boiling point components (such as inorganic salts), which may damage the injection port and chromatography column. Therefore, for an unknown sample, we should estimate the components and the boiling range of the sample. If the sample is simple, the sample components can be vaporized for direct analysis. If there are components that cannot be directly analyzed by gas chromatography in the sample, or if the sample concentration is too low, it is necessary to carry out the pretreatment method, such as adsorption, resolution, extraction, concentration, dilution, purification, derivatization, etc.

6. 2 Equipment configuration of GC

The equipment configuration should take them consideration that the separation and detection conditions based on the analytes, such as sampling device, carrier gas, column and detector.

Generally, the detector type should be determined first. FID detector is often chosen for the hydrocarbons; ECD detector are always used for substances with more negative electron groups (F, Cl, etc.) and less hydrocarbon; TCD detector is general selected for the analytes with low sensitivity or containing non – hydrocarbons; FPD detector is for samples containing sulfur and phosphorus.

Column is selected according to the nature of the components. Non – polar column is selected for separating non – polar substances and polar column is adopted for separating polar substances. After the column is determined, the working temperature of the column is determined according to the difference of the partition coefficient of the components being examined. Simple system adopts the isothermal method, and the complex system with large difference of the distribution coefficients is analyzed by the temperature programming.

Carrier gases such as hydrogen, nitrogen and helium, are commonly used. Hydrogen and helium are often used as the carrier gas for packed column chromatography due to the small molecular weight. Nitrogen is often used as the carrier gas for capillary gas chromatography because of their large molecular. The gas chromategraphy mass spectrometry uses helium as the carrier gas.

6.3 Optimization of GC separation conditions

Separation can be attempted after sample preparation and equipment configuration. The initial separation conditions mainly include the injection volume, the inlet temperature, the detector temperature, the column temperature, and the flow rate of carrier gas. The injection volume is determined by the sample concentration, the column capacity, and the detector sensitivity. The injection volume of the packed column is usually $1 \sim 5\mu l$ when the sample concentration is less than 10mg/ml. Generally, the injection volume is less than $2\mu l$ for the capillary column. The inlet temperature is primarily determined by the boiling point range of the sample, as well as the operation temperature of column. In principle, the higher inlet temperature is good for sample vaporization in a certain range, which is generally close to the highest boiling point of the component in the sample but lower than the degradation temperature. The column temperature is the key factor influencing the separation in gas chromatography, which should be optimized according to the nature of analytes and the different separation purpose. Each column has its maximum temperature and the operation column temperature should be no more than the maximum. The flow rate of carrier gas should be set according to the type of column. Splitting device is used for the capillary column, allowing relatively low flow rate no more than 6ml/min. Higher flow rate can be adopted for the packed column.

The purpose of the separation condition optimization is to achieve the desired separation result in the shortest analysis time. When changing the column temperature and the carrier gas flowrate cannot achieve the purpose of baseline separation, the longer columns and even columns with different stationary phases should be used because column is critical for separation in gas chromatography.

6.4 Quantitative method in GC

Quantitative methods for GC include the peak area normalization method, the internal standard method, the external standard method and the standard addition method. The peak area normalization method is the simplest but the least accurate, which is optional only if the sample consists of homologues or only for the rough estimation. The external standard method means that the sample solution and the reference solution are injected into the chromatography system and the peak area of the analyte is measured for the quantification. The internal standard method is quantified with the response ratio between the analyte and the internal standard. The internal standard is added to the standard sample and the unknown sample respectively, which can offset the error caused by fluctuations of operation conditions (including injection volume). As for the standard addition method, a certain amount of standard substance is added to the sample and the content is calculated by the increase of peak area. The standard addition method is a special quantitative method in the headspace – GC to diminish the matrix effect.

实验三 顶空进样气相色谱法测定藿香正气水中乙醇的含量

扫码"学一学"

【实验目的】

1. 学习气相色谱法中顶空进样法的原理。
2. 学习色谱法测定药用辅料含量的流程。
3. 学习顶空气相色谱条件的建立与优化。

【实验原理】

1. 藿香正气水组成及其制法 藿香正气水，来源于宋代《太平惠民和剂局方》的藿香正气散，由苍术、陈皮、厚朴（姜制）、白芷、茯苓、大腹皮、生半夏、甘草浸膏、广藿香油和紫苏叶油十味中药或其提取物组成，具有解表化湿，理气和中的功效；主要用于外感风寒、内伤湿滞或夏伤暑湿所致的感冒，症见头痛昏重、胸膈痞闷、脘腹胀痛、呕吐泄泻；胃肠型感冒见上述证候者。藿香正气水为中药酊剂，制备时将苍术、陈皮、厚朴、白芷分别用60%乙醇作溶剂，浸渍24小时后进行渗漉，得到渗漉液；茯苓加水煮沸后，80℃温浸取汁；生半夏用冷水浸泡至透心后，加干姜并加水煎煮二次；大腹皮加水煎煮，甘草浸膏打碎后水煮化开；将上述提取液合并，滤过，滤液浓缩至适量。最后将广藿香油、紫苏叶油用乙醇适量溶解后与以上溶液混匀，用乙醇与水适量调整乙醇含量，静置，滤过，灌装，即得。由此可见，乙醇不仅作为主要的提取溶剂，而且是制剂中的主要溶媒。《中国药典》（2020年版）一部中规定，藿香正气水需要进行乙醇量检查，结果应在40% ~ 50%。

2. 顶空进样的原理 顶空进样法是指将样品溶液置于密闭小瓶中，在恒温控制的加热室中进行加热，至挥发性组分在液态和气态达到平衡后，由顶空进样器吸取一定体积的上方气体注入色谱系统中。该方式适用于样品溶液中挥发性组分的分离和测定，可以消除不挥发药物基质对进样口和色谱柱的污染。其分析过程包括加热平衡、取样、进样和气相色谱分析。根据取样方式不同，顶空进样可以分为静态顶空进样和动态顶空进样两种方式，在药物分析中主要使用前者。

图3 – 1为静态顶空进样瓶示意图，供试品溶液装载在顶空进样瓶内，密封置于加热室中，恒温一段时间后，挥发性的待测成分在供试品溶液与上层气相之间达到平衡。假设供试品溶液中待测成分的浓度为 C_0，供试品溶液体积为 V_s，上层气相体积为 V_g，平衡后溶液中样品浓度为 C_s，气相中样品浓度为 C_g，则：

$$C_0 V_s = C_s V_s + C_g V_g = K C_g V_s + C_g V_g$$

$$C_0 = K C_g + \frac{C_g V_g}{V_s} = K C_g + \beta C_g = (K + \beta) C_g$$

其中 K 为分配系数，等于待测成分在溶液中和气相中的浓度比，β 为相比率，等于气相体积与溶液体积之比。对于密闭的顶空进样瓶，当温度一定时，K 和 β 均为常数，供试品中待测组分浓度与其上方气相中的浓度成正比。

顶空进样装置主要包括顶空进样瓶、恒温装置和取样进样装置。顶空进样瓶一般为10ml 或 20ml 的玻璃瓶，具有硅橡胶隔垫密封。恒温装置可以设定温度和时间。取样进样装置由取样针、定量环、转移管等组成，可以定量的将供试品溶液上方的气体注入气相色谱仪。

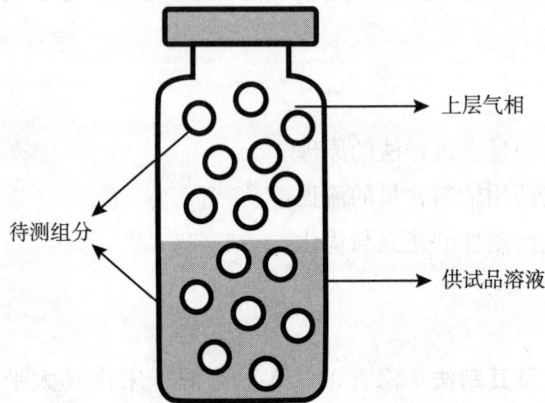

图 3 - 1 　静态顶空进样瓶示意图

【仪器与试剂】

1. 仪器　气相色谱仪，FID 检测器，顶空进样器，高纯氮气，氢气，空气，分析天平，量瓶（100ml）、移液管（1ml、5ml）、气相手动进样针（1μl）。

2. 试剂　藿香正气水（市售品，含乙醇40% ~ 50%）；无水乙醇（纯度 >99.8%）；正丙醇（密度为 0.83g/cm³）。

【实验内容】

1. 对照品溶液的配制　取无水乙醇 1.0g，精密称定，置100ml 量瓶中，精密加入内标正丙醇 1ml，加水稀释至刻度，摇匀，作为对照品溶液。

2. 供试品溶液的配制　精密量取藿香正气水 2ml，置100ml 量瓶中，精密加入内标正丙醇 1ml，加水稀释至刻度，摇匀，作为供试品溶液。

3. 色谱条件设置　色谱柱：DB - WAX 熔融石英毛细管柱（30m ×0.32mm ×0.1μm）；载气：氮气；柱内流量：4ml/min；柱温：60℃；进样口温度：190℃，检测器温度：220℃；FID检测条件：燃气为氢气，设定流速30ml/min，助燃气为空气，设定流速300ml/min。直接进样体积为 1μl，分流比 1∶20。顶空进样加热温度为 70℃，加热平衡时间为 20min，传输线温度为110℃，进样体积为 1ml，分流比 1∶5。色谱系统适用性试验要求，按乙醇计算理论塔板数不得低于300，在此条件下乙醇与内标峰的分离度应大于 2。

4. 直接进样法测定含量　精密量取 1μl 对照品溶液注入气相色谱仪，记录色谱图，以乙醇与正丙醇的峰面积，计算校正因子。精密量取 1μl 供试品溶液注入气相色谱仪，记录色谱图，按内标法以乙醇与正丙醇的峰面积比值计算供试品中乙醇的含量。

5. 顶空进样法测定含量　精密量取对照品溶液 5ml 置于 20ml 顶空进样瓶内，立即盖好瓶盖，压紧密封，放入顶空进样器内进样，记录色谱图，以乙醇与正丙醇的峰面积，计算校正因子。精密量取供试品溶液 5ml 置于 20ml 顶空进样瓶内，立即盖好瓶盖，压紧密封，放入顶空进样器内进样，记录色谱图，按内标法以乙醇与丙醇的峰面积比值计算供试品中乙醇的含量。

【数据记录与处理】

1. 对照品溶液的配制记录

表 3-1　对照品溶液的配制记录

对照品的称样量	对照品溶液浓度（mg/ml）	内标的计算量	内标溶液的浓度（mg/ml）

2. 含量测定原始数据

表 3-2　溶液直接进样数据记录

		乙醇			正丙醇		
		保留时间（min）	峰面积	平均峰面积	保留时间（min）	峰面积	平均峰面积
对照品	1						
	2						
	3						
供试品	1						
	2						
	3						

表 3-3　顶空进样数据记录

		乙醇			正丙醇		
		保留时间（min）	峰面积	平均峰面积	保留时间（min）	峰面积	平均峰面积
对照品	1						
	2						
	3						
供试品	1						
	2						
	3						

3. 校正因子的计算　根据校正因子（f）计算公式：

$$f = (A_S / C_S) / (A_R / C_R)$$

计算每次对照品溶液进样分析所得的校正因子 f，并计算三次进样得到的校正因子平均值 $f_{均}$（其中 A_R 和 C_R 分别代表对照品的峰面积和浓度；A_S 和 C_S 分别代表内标的峰面积和浓度）。

表 3-4 校正因子的计算结果

	1	2	3	平均值
直接进样校正因子（f）				
顶空进样校正因子（f）				

4. 含量计算 根据含量计算公式：

$$乙醇含量（\%）= \frac{f \cdot A_R \cdot D}{(A_S' / C_S')} \cdot 100\%$$

计算藿香正气水中乙醇的含量（其中 A_S' 和 C_S' 分别代表供试品溶液中内标的峰面积和浓度；A_R 代表供试品溶液中乙醇的峰面积；D 代表供试品的稀释倍数）。

表 3-5 乙醇含量的计算结果

	1	2	3	平均值
直接进样测定乙醇含量（%）				
顶空进样测定乙醇含量（%）				

【实验讨论与指导】

1. 测定藿香正气水中乙醇含量的原因 从藿香正气水的制剂工艺中可以看出，乙醇不仅是该复方主要化学成分的提取溶剂，而且是该制剂中的主要药用辅料，用于保持制剂的均匀状态。如果乙醇含量过低，部分化学成分可能析出，形成沉淀，影响药效；如果乙醇含量过高，虽然保持了液体制剂稳定的状态，但会造成使用者摄入更多的乙醇，引发不安全因素。因此《中国药典》（2020 年版）一部中规定，藿香正气水需要进行乙醇量检查，结果应在 40% ~ 50%。

2. 气相色谱中进样方式的选择 直接进样是气相色谱中常用的进样方式，样品中所有的物质都会进入气相色谱仪，会存在一些杂质，因此对色谱分离带来一定影响。未处理干净的样品长时间分析后，可能会堵塞进样针或者色谱柱。

顶空进样方式适用于易挥发的待测组分。待测组分和样品基质的沸点不同，在加热状态下，待测组分挥发实现了预先的物理分离；随后再将较为干净的顶空气体进样分析，其背景干扰较小。由于需要对顶空进样瓶进行加热平衡，因此该进样方式的分析时间较直接进样长，并且平衡时间长短也直接影响了分析方法的重复性。另外进样的是平衡后的顶空气体，所以进样量一般较大，具有更高的灵敏度。

因此在进样方式选择时候，首先可以根据待测成分的性质和样品基质的复杂程度进行合理选择，沸点低的待测组分选择顶空进样，沸点高的则选择直接进样；其次需要考虑待测成分的含量，在色谱条件一致的情况下，选择能够实现高灵敏度检测的进样方式；最后综合考虑方法的重复性和加热平衡时间。

3. 顶空进样的注意事项

（1）顶空进样瓶中的液体量不宜太多，以免污染到取样针；在待测成分灵敏度可以满足的情况下，尽量选择较少的溶液体积。

（2）选择合适的溶剂溶解样品，对于水溶性的药物，一般选择水作为溶剂；对于水不溶药物，可以选择二甲亚砜等适宜的有机溶剂溶解，所选择的溶剂不得干扰待测成分的检测。

（3）顶空加热温度应适宜，可以通过考察加热温度和待测成分峰面积响应之间的关系，确定加热温度；同时加热温度应小于溶剂沸点，防止溶剂的挥发影响到顶空进样瓶上的蒸气压而影响进样的重复性。

（4）装样后立刻用顶空瓶盖盖好，压紧。在进样之前，应该充分的震荡顶空进样瓶，使乙醇能充分挥发；同时应充分考察顶空加热时间，保证待测组分充分挥发到顶空瓶上方空气中，保证进样的重复性。

（5）传输线温度应高于顶空加热温度，防止待测组分取样后在取样器内重新冷凝，影响色谱分析。

Experiment 3   Determination of Ethanol in Huoxiang Zhengqi Shui by Headspace – Gas Chromatography

1. Experimental purposes

1. 1 To learn the basic principle of headspace – gas chromatography.

1. 2 To learn theprocedures for the determination of the pharmaceutical excipient by chromatography method.

1. 3 To learn development and optimization of headspace – gas chromatography.

2. Experimental principles

2. 1 The composition and preparation of Huoxiang Zhengqi Shui

Huoxiang Zhengqi Shui, a tincture of herbal formula was derived from a powder formula Huoxiang Zhengqi San recorded in a medicine book named Taiping Huimin Heji Jufang in the Song Dynasty. The formula is composed of Atractylodis Rhizoma, Citri Reticulatae Pericarpium, Magnoliae Officinalis Cortex (processed with ginger), Angelicae Dahuricae Radix, Arecae Pericarpium, Poria, Pinelliae Rhizoma, Licorice Extract, Patchouli Oil and Perillae Folium Oil, which could release the exterior and resolve dampness, and regulate the flow of qi to harmonize the middle – energizer. Its indications include cold due to affliction from external wind – cold and internal retention of dampness or summer – heat and dampness, with manifestation of headache with heavey sensation, constriction in the chest, distending pain in the stomach and abdomen, vomiting and diarrhea, gastrointestinal cold with above symptoms. The preparation of the tincture is as follows: Atractylodis Rhizoma, Citri Reticulatae Pericarpium, Magnoliae Officinalis Cortex (processed with ginger) and Angelicae Dahuricae Radix is macerated separately for 24h using 60% ethanol as solvent and then extracted by percolation process to produce extract. Poria is heated with water to boiling and macerated at 80℃. Pinelliae Rhizoma is macerated with cold water until softened thoroughly and decocted with water for two times after adding the dried ginger. Arecae Pericarpium is decocted with water and Licorice Extract is pulverized and dissolved in boiling water. The above decoctions and filter are combined and concentrated properly. Patchouli Oil and Perillae Folium Oil are dissolved in a quantity of ethanol and mixed with the above solutions well. The mixture is adjusted with ethanol and water to a certain ethanol content, allowing to stand, filter and pack. From the procedure, it can be seen that ethanol is not only the main extraction solvent, but also the main liquid in which the components of the herb medicine are dissolved. The Chinese Pharmacopoeia 2020 edition requires that Huoxiang Zhengqi Shui needs to be tested for ethanol conten with 40% ~ 50%.

2. 2 The principle of headspace – gas chromatography (HS – GC)

The sample solution is placed in a sealed vial and heated by a thermostatic heating device. When the equilibrium of the volatile component between gas phase and liquid phase reached, an aliquot of this vapor – phase mixture is withdrawn by headspace sampler and transferred to the gas chromatography system for the separation and analysis. This method is called headspace – gas chromatography (HS – GC) and suitable for the separation of volatile components in sample solutions because headspace sampling can reduce the contamination of nonvolatile drug matrix in GC injector and column. The procedures of HS – GC include the heating and equilibrium, the sampling, the transferring to injector and the separation in gas chromatography. According to the difference in the sampling method, there are static headspace mode and dynamic headspace mode and the former mode is usually applied in the pharmaceutical analysis.

Fig. 3 – 1 shows a schematic representation of a vial used in static headspace mode. The vial containing the sample solution is sealed and placed in the heater for the equilibrium. After a certain time, the volatile analytes, originally present in the sample phase, are distributed between the sample phase and the upper gaseous phase at equilibrium. This is the foundation relationship between the concentration of the initial analyte in liquid phase (C_0) and that of the analyte in the gas phase (C_g). V_S is the volume of the sample solution. V_g is the volume of the gaseous phase. C_S is the analyte concentration in the sample phase after equilibrium.

$$C_0 V_S = C_S V_S + C_g V_g = K C_g V_S + C_g V_g$$

$$C_0 = K C_g + \frac{C_g V_g}{V_S} = K C_g + \beta C_g = (K + \beta) C_g$$

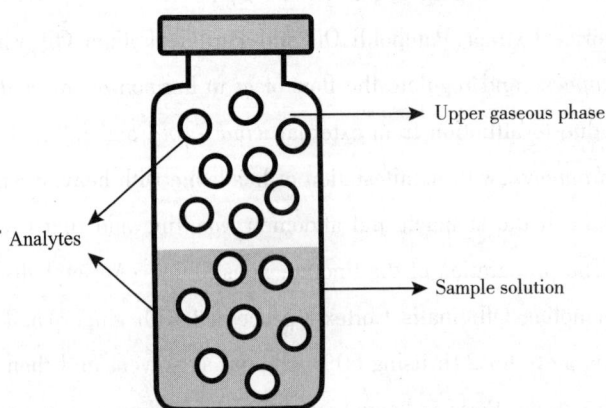

Fig. 3 – 1   Schematic representation of a vial used in static headspace sampling

K is partition coefficient and defined as the ratio of the concentration of the analyte in the sample phase to that of the analyte in the gaseous phase. β is the phase ratio and defined as the ratio of the volume of the gaseous phase to that of the sample liquid phase. For a certain analyte in a sealed container, whose K and β are constant after equilibrating the vial to the desired temperature condition, illustrating the c_0 is clearly proportional to C_s.

The headspace sampler apparatus includes sealed vials, heater for equilibrium and sampler for injection. The volume of sealed vial is about 10ml or 20ml with the silicone rubber. The heater could be set the temperature and time for equilibrating the vial. The sampling portion includes a syringe, sample loop and transfer line, which could withdraw and transfer quantitatively an aliquot of the headspace within a vial to a gas chromatography system.

3. Apparatus and Reagents

3. 1 Apparatus

Gas chromatography system; Flame ionization detector (FID); High purity nitrogen; Hydrogen; Air; Analytical balance; Volumetric flask (100ml); Transfer pipettes (1ml); Manual injection syringe for GC (1μl).

3. 2 Reagents

Huoxiang Zhengqi Shui (commercial products, containing ethanol 40% ~ 50%); Ethanol reference substance (purity is more than 99. 8%); n – propanol (density:0. 83g/cm^3).

4. Experimental contents

4. 1 Preparation of the reference solution

Accurately weigh 1. 0g of ethanol reference substance and pipette 1ml of n – octanol to a 100ml volumetric flask, then dissolve them with water to the mark and shake well before use.

4. 2 Preparation of the sample solution

Accurately pipette 2ml of the sample solution and 1ml of n – propanol reference substance to a 100ml volumetric flask, then add water to the mark and shake well before use.

4. 3 Setting of gas chromatography conditions

Afused silica DB – WAX capillary column (30m ×0. 32mm ×1. 0μm)or similar columns is used as the stationary phase. The carrier gas is nitrogen. The column flow is about 4ml/min. The column temperature is set at 60℃. The inlet temperature and hydrogen flame detector temperature are 190℃ and 220℃, respectively. A hydrogen with the flow rate of 30ml/min is used in the FID and the air is used as assistant gas at the flow rate of 300ml/min.

The injection volume is set at 1μl with the split ratio of 1 : 20 in the direct injection mode. In headspace sampling mode, sample equilibration temperature is set at 70℃ for equilibration time of 20min. The transfer line temperature is set at 110℃. The injection volume is set at 1ml with the split ratio of 1 : 5.

Chromatographic system suitability requires the number of theoretical plates of the column is not less than 300, calculated with the reference of the peak of ethanol. The resolution between ethanol and the internal standard is more than 2.

4. 4 Determination of ethanol by direct injection

Inject 1μl of the reference solution into the gas chromatography system and record the peak area of ethanol and n – propanol to calculate the correction factor.

Inject $1\,\mu l$ of the sample solution and record the peak area of ethanol and n – propanol to calculate the content of ethanol in sample by the internal standard method.

4. 5 Determination of ethanol by headspace sampling mode

Pipette 5ml of the reference solution to a 20ml vial and seal the cap quickly followed by being tighten. Place the vial in the heater for equilibrium and injection. Record the peak area of the ethanol and n – propanol, respectively, and calculate the correction factor.

Pipette 5ml of the sample solution to a 20ml vial and seal the cap quickly followed by being tighten. Place the vial in the heater for equilibrium and injection. Record the peak area of the ethanol and n – propanol, respectively, and calculate the content using the internal method.

5. Data record and processing

5. 1 Record for the preparation of the reference solution

Table 3 – 1   Record for the preparation of the reference solution

Amount of the reference standard	Concentration of the reference standard (mg/ml)	Amount of the internal standard	Concentration of the internal standard (mg/ml)

5. 2 Original data for determination

Table 3 – 2   Original data for determination in direct injection mode

		Ethanol			n – propanol		
		Retention time (min)	Peak area	Average of peak area	Retention time (min)	Peak area	Average of peak area
Reference Standard	1						
	2						
	3						
Sample	1						
	2						
	3						

Table 3 – 3   Original data for determination in headspace sampling mode

		Ethanol			n – propanol		
		Retention time (min)	Peak area	Average of peak area	Retention time (min)	Peak area	Average of peak area
Reference Standard	1						
	2						
	3						
Sample	1						
	2						
	3						

5. 3 Calculation of the correction factor

Calculate the correction factor (f) according to the following equation:

$$f = (A_S / C_S) / (A_R / C_R)$$

and repeat three times to obtain the average value f_{ave} (A_R and C_R represent the peak area and concentration of the reference standard, respectively. A_S and C_S represent the peak area and concentration of the internal standard, respectively).

Table 3 – 4 The calculation results of the correction factor

	1	2	3	f_{ave}
f (Direct injection)				
f (Headspace sampling)				

5. 4 Calculation of the percentage of ethanol in sample

Calculate the concentration of ethanol in the sample solution according to the following equation:

$$Ethanol\ percentage(\%) = \frac{f \cdot A_R \cdot D}{(A_S' / C_S')} \cdot 100\%$$

(A_S' and C_S' represent the peak area and concentration of the internal standard in sample, respectively. A_R represent the peak area of ethanol in sample. D is the dilute multiple during the preparation of the sample solution).

Table 3 – 5 The result of the percentage of ethanol in sample

	1	2	3	Average
Percentage (%) by direct injection				
Percentage (%) by headspace sampling				

6. Discussion and guidance

6. 1 The reason for the determination of the ethanol content in Huoxiang Zhengqi Shui

The preparation process of Huoxiang Zhengqi Shui shows that ethanol is not only the main extraction solvent extracting chemical components of the formula, but also the main pharmaceutical excipient in the preparation for maintaining the uniform state. If the ethanol content was too low, some chemical components might be precipitated, which could affect the efficacy. While the more ethanol content might lead to excessive ethanol intake with uncertainly harm, despite the more stability of the chemical components. Therefore, the Chinese Pharmacopoeia 2020 edition requires that Huoxiang Zhengqi Shui needs to be tested for ethanol content with 40% ~ 50%.

6. 2 Selection of the injection mode in GC

Direct injection solution is a common injection mode in the gas chromatography, which allows all the components in the sample to enter the gas chromatograph with some possible impurities, influencing the chromatographic separation such as blocking the syringe or column with the untreated sample after long time run.

The headspace sampling is applicable to analysis of the volatile components. Due to the different boiling points between the analytes and the matrix, the analytes will vaporize in the upper gaseous phase, achieving the physical separation firstly and then the neat vapor phase in headspace will be sampled and injected for gas chromatographic separation with little interfered background. The headspace sampling mode spends longer time than the direct injection mode because of the heating for equilibrium, which will affect the repeatability of the analysis. In addition, the injection volume of the headspace vapor is generally larger resulting in higher sensitivity.

When selecting the injection mode, the character of the analytes and the complexity of the sample matrix should be considered. The headspace sampling is suitable for the analytes with low boiling point and the direct injection for those with high boiling point. And content of the analytes should be taken into accounted for the selection of the proper injection mode, achieving high sensitivity under the same chromatographic conditions. Also, the repeatability of the analysis and the heating equilibrium time should be allowed for comprehensively.

6.3 Precautions for headspace sampling

a. The amount of liquid in the vial should not be unreasonably much for avoiding the contamination of the sampling needle. If the sensitivity of detection on the component could be satisfied, a smaller solution volume might be the best.

b. A suitable solvent should be selected to dissolve the sample. For water - soluble analytes, water is generally selected and for water - insoluble analytes, suitable organic solvent should be considered such as dimethyl sulfoxide. The selected solvent must not interfere with the detection of the analytes.

c. The heating temperature should be suitable. which can be determined by examining the relationship between the heating temperature and the response of the analytes. The heating temperature should be less than the boiling point of the solvent to prevent the evaporation of the solvent, which might affect the vapor pressure in the sealed vial, changing the repeatability of the injection.

d. Immediately the vial should be capped tightly after being loaded the sample. Before the injection, the vial should be mixed to improve the transfer of volatile ethanol from the sample into the headspace of the vial. The heating time should be investigated to ensure that the analytes are fully volatilized into the headspace for the good repeatability of the injection.

e. The temperature of the transfer line should be higher than the equilibrium temperature to prevent the analytes in the vapor phase being condensed again in the sampler, which will affect the chromatographic analysis.

实验四　程序升温气相色谱法测定盐酸阿米替林中的残留溶剂

【实验目的】

1. 学习气相色谱程序升温法的特点及优势。

2. 学习气相色谱法测定药物中残留溶剂的流程。

3. 学习程序升温法的设计原理。

扫码"看一看"

【实验原理】

1. 盐酸阿米替林中的残留溶剂限度　药品中的残留溶剂是指在生产原料、辅料或制剂的过程中使用或产生的挥发性有机化合物。它们在生产过程中若未能全部清除，服用后将对人体会产生毒性或致癌作用。《中国药典》和人用药物注册技术要求国际协调会（ICH）均对常见残留溶剂的限度进行了规定。

盐酸阿米替林（图 4-1）是一种三环类的抗抑郁药，主要用于治疗焦虑性或激动性抑郁症。盐酸阿米替林是由二苯并环庚二烯酮经加成、消除、成盐而得的产品。第一步加成、消除反应所用溶剂为四氢呋喃和乙醚，得到产物用甲苯多次萃取得羟基阿米替林粗品，然后与盐酸成盐，最后用异丙醇和活性炭加热回流提纯精制得盐酸阿米替林粉末。由此可见，盐酸阿米替林的生产和精制过程中使用了四氢呋喃、乙醚、甲苯、异丙醇等有机溶剂，其中乙醚由于沸点低，在最后一步的加热回流中几乎挥发干净。但四氢呋喃、甲苯、异丙醇并不能保证完全清除，这些二、三类溶剂对人体和环境存在潜在的毒性，因此根据《中国药典》（2020 年版）盐酸阿米替林中的残留溶剂限度为：甲苯 $\leqslant 0.089\%$；异丙醇 $\leqslant 0.5\%$，四氢呋喃 $\leqslant 0.072\%$。

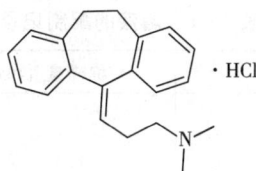

图 4-1　盐酸阿米替林的结构

2. 程序升温法的原理　气相色谱法分离多个不同性质的待测物时，如果色谱分离保持在较低温度，往往洗脱的前几个色谱峰峰形良好，时间适宜，但是高沸点成分则会与固定相作用时间增加，从而出峰延迟并峰形展宽。如果提高柱温，这些高沸点成分在固定相和流动相中的作用加快，更快地从色谱柱洗脱，但是低沸点的组分可能在色谱柱中没有足够保留。在遇到这种问题时，常需要采用程序升温法。

程序升温法是指在一个气相色谱分析周期内，色谱柱的温度按设置的程序连续地随时间线性或非线性逐渐升高，使不同沸点的组分在适宜的温度下分离的技术。采用程序升温法，逐渐提高柱温，既保证低沸点成分获得良好的分离，又使得高沸点成分能够较快得被洗脱，加速整个色谱分离过程，获得峰形良好的色谱峰。由于气相色谱法是残留溶剂测定的常用方法，而药品中残留溶剂种类较多，且沸点相差较大，因此常采用程序升温气相色谱法进行分析。

【仪器与试剂】

1. 仪器　气相色谱仪，FID 检测器，高纯氮气，氢气，空气，分析天平，微量注射器（10μl），量瓶（100ml、25ml），移液管（1ml、2ml）。

2. 试剂　盐酸阿米替林原料药（纯度大于 99%）；甲苯、异丙醇、四氢呋喃和二甲基甲酰胺均为分析纯试剂。

【实验内容】

1. 对照品溶液的配制　取甲苯、四氢呋喃与异丙醇适量，精密称定，用二甲基甲酰胺稀释制成每1ml中约含甲苯17.8μg、四氢呋喃14.4μg与异丙醇100μg的混合溶液，作为对照品溶液。

2. 供试品溶液的配制　取盐酸阿米替林原料药适量，精密称定，加二甲基甲酰胺溶解并稀释制成每1ml中约含盐酸阿米替林20mg的溶液，作为供试品溶液。

3. 色谱条件的设置　色谱柱：以6%氰丙基苯基-94%二甲基聚硅氧烷为固定液的毛细管柱（30m×0.25mm×0.25μm）或同类型色谱柱；载气：氮气；柱内流量：4ml/min，分流比1:20；进样口温度：250℃；FID检测器温度：250℃。采用程序升温法：色谱柱温起始温度80℃，维持10分钟，以每分钟20℃的速率升温至200℃，维持5分钟。

4. 残留溶剂测定　取对照品溶液1μl注入气相色谱仪，各成分峰间的分离度均应符合要求；再精密量取供试品溶液与对照品溶液各1μl，分别注入气相色谱仪，记录色谱图，按外标法以峰面积计算，甲苯、四氢呋喃与异丙醇的残留量均应符合规定。

【数据记录和处理】

1. 溶液的配制记录

表4-1　溶液的配制记录

溶液		称样量（m）	溶液浓度（C）
对照品溶液	四氢呋喃		
	异丙醇		
	甲苯		
供试品溶液	盐酸阿米替林		

2. 溶剂残留测定的原始数据

表4-2　溶剂残留测定的原始数据

	序号	峰面积（A）			分离度（R）	
		四氢呋喃	异丙醇	甲苯	四氢呋喃-异丙醇	异丙醇-甲苯
对照品溶液	1					
	2					
	3					
供试品溶液	1					
	2					
	3					

注：甲苯沸点110.6℃，异丙醇沸点82℃，四氢呋喃沸点65.4℃

3. 残留溶剂的测定结果

根据外标法公式：$C_X = (A_X/A_R) \cdot C_R$，计算供试品溶液中残留溶剂的浓度。式中：$C_X$为供试品溶液中残留溶剂浓度；$C_R$为残留溶剂对照品浓度；$A_X$为供试品溶液中残留溶剂峰面积；$A_R$为残留溶剂对照品峰面积。根据供试品溶液中残留溶剂的浓度与供试品的浓度（20mg/ml）百分比计算盐酸阿米替林中的溶剂残留量。

表 4 – 3　残留溶剂测定结果

	含量（%）		
	四氢呋喃	异丙醇	甲苯
第一次			
第二次			
第三次			
平均值			

【实验讨论与指导】

1. 残留溶剂及限度要求　根据《中国药典》（2020 年版）规定：药品中常见的残留溶剂及限度要求见下表，除另有规定，第一、第二、第三类溶剂的残留限度应符合下表。对其他溶剂，应根据生产工艺特点，制定相应的限度，使其符合产品规范、药品生产质量管理规范（GMP）或其他基本的质量要求。新药报批和注册，对于溶剂残留的要求参照 ICH 要求执行。

表 4 – 4　药品中常见的溶剂残留及限度

第一类溶剂（应该避免使用）		第二类溶剂（应该限制使用）		第三类溶剂（GMP 或其他质量要求限制使用）		第四类溶剂（尚无足够毒理学资料）	
溶剂名称	限度（%）	溶剂名称	限度（%）	溶剂名称	限度（%）	溶剂名称	限度（%）
苯	0.0002	乙腈	0.041	乙酸	0.5	1, 1 – 二乙氧基丙烷	
四氯化碳	0.0004	氯苯	0.036	丙酮	0.5	1, 1 – 二甲氧基甲烷	
1, 2 – 二氯乙烷	0.0005	三氯甲烷	0.006	甲氧基苯	0.5	2, 2 – 二甲氧基丙烷	
1, 1 – 二氯乙烯	0.0008	环己烷	0.388	正丁醇	0.5	异辛烷	
1, 1, 1 – 三氯乙烷	0.15	1, 2 – 二氯乙烯	0.187	仲丁醇	0.5	异丙醚	
		二氯甲烷	0.06	乙酸丁酯	0.5	甲基异丙基酮	
		1, 2 – 二甲氧基乙烷	0.01	叔丁基甲基醚	0.5	甲基四氢呋喃	
		N, N – 二甲基乙酰胺	0.109	异丙基苯	0.5	石油醚	
		N, N – 二甲基甲酰胺	0.088	二甲基亚砜	0.5	三氯乙酸	
		二氧六环	0.038	乙醇	0.5	三氟乙酸	
		2 – 乙氧基乙醇	0.016	乙酸乙酯	0.5		
		乙二醇	0.062	乙醚	0.5		
		甲酰胺	0.022	甲酸乙酯	0.5		
		正己烷	0.029	甲酸	0.5		
		甲醇	0.300	正庚烷	0.5		
		2 – 甲氧基乙醇	0.005	乙酸异丁酯	0.5		
		甲基丁基酮	0.005	乙酸异丙酯	0.5		

第一类溶剂 （应该避免使用）		第二类溶剂 （应该限制使用）		第三类溶剂 （GMP 或其他 质量要求限制使用）		第四类溶剂 （尚无足够毒理学资料）	
溶剂名称	限度 （%）	溶剂名称	限度 （%）	溶剂名称	限度 （%）	溶剂名称	限度 （%）
		甲基环己烷	0.118	乙酸甲酯	0.5		
		N-甲基吡咯烷酮	0.053	3-甲基-1-丁醇	0.5		
		硝基甲烷	0.005	丁酮	0.5		
		吡啶	0.02	甲基异丁基酮	0.5		
		四氢噻吩	0.016	异丁醇	0.5		
		四氢化萘	0.01	正戊烷	0.5		
		四氢呋喃	0.072	正戊醇	0.5		
		甲苯	0.089	正丙醇	0.5		
		1，1，2-三氯乙烯	0.008	异丙醇	0.5		
		二甲苯	0.217	乙酸丙酯	0.5		

2. 程序升温的升温方式 程序升温是气相色谱分析中一项常用且十分重要的技术，对于组分复杂、沸程较宽样品，必须采用合适的程序升温方式，分别满足样品中各个组分的最佳柱温要求。实际中，普遍使用线性升温方式，可分一阶线性程序升温和 N 阶线性程序升温。在气相色谱分析中，对于组分沸点范围较宽、化学性质类似的样品（如同系物），可选用一阶线性升温；样品组分沸点范围很宽、性质差异大，应选择 N 阶程序升温，N 的确定应根据化合物的多少、需要达到的分离效果、仪器的条件等各方面来选择。程序升温中，一定要在一个温度程序执行完成后，需等待色谱仪回到初始状态并稳定后，才能进行下一次进样。

3. 残留溶剂测定的进样方式 顶空进样是残留溶剂测定中最常用的进样方式，由于大部分残留溶剂沸点较低，因此可以通过加热密闭顶空瓶中的样品溶液，对顶空瓶中蒸气相中的有机挥发性成分进行气相色谱分析。对于水溶性较好的药物通常以水为溶剂，对于非水溶性药物，可采用二甲基甲酰胺、二甲亚砜等沸点较高的溶剂；根据供试品和待测溶剂的溶解度，选择适宜的萃取溶剂且应不干扰待测溶剂的测定。顶空进样的方式能够排除或减少药物基质对进样口的污染和色谱分离的干扰，且灵敏度也高于直接进样的方式，因此已成为药物中残留溶剂测定的首选方法，但该方式需要配备专门的顶空进样装置。

直接进样法主要用于沸点较高的残留溶剂，如二甲基甲酰胺、二甲亚砜、N-甲基咯烷酮等，此类高沸点溶剂用顶空进样测定的灵敏度不如直接进样，一般不宜用顶空进样方式测定，应采用溶液直接进样法测定。在未配置顶空进样装置时亦可采用直接进样法对低沸点溶剂进行测定。直接进样法的主要不足是多次进样后，进样口容易受到药品基质的影响。

Experiment 4   Determination of Residual Solvents in Amitriptyline Hydrochloride by Temperature Programming Gas Chromatography

1. Experimental purposes

1. 1 To learn the advantage of temperature programming gas chromatography.

1. 2 To learn the procedures for the determination of residual solvents in drug substances by gas chromatography.

1. 3 To learn the design principle of temperature programming.

2. Experimental principles

2. 1 The limits of residual solvents in amitriptyline hydrochloride

Residual solvents in pharmaceuticals are volatile organic compounds used or produced during the production of active pharmaceutical ingredients, pharmaceutical excipients and pharmaceutical preparations. If they are not completely removed during the production process, they will have toxic or carcinogenic effects on the human body after taking. Therefore, their residue in drug substances should be controlled at low limits according to the Chinese Pharmacopoeia or the International Coordination Committee (ICH).

Amitriptyline hydrochloride (Fig. 4 – 1) is a tricyclic antidepressant and mainly used for anxiety or agitated depression. It is prepared by the addition, elimination and salt formation of diphenyl cycloheptadienone. In the first step, tetrahydrofuran and ether are used as solvents for addition and elimination reaction. The product is extracted by toluene for several times to obtain hydroxy amitriptyline crude products, and then form into salt with hydrochloric acid. Finally, the powder of amitriptyline hydrochloride was purified by refluxing with isopropanol and activated carbon. It can be known that tetrahydrofuran, ethyl ether, toluene and isopropanol are involved during the synthesis of amitriptyline hydrochloride. Therefore, the residue of these organic solvents in amitriptyline hydrochloride should be controlled except ethyl ether due to its low boiling point. Tetrahydrofuran, toluene and isopropanol belong to the second or third category of solvents and they have potential toxicity to human body and environment. According to the 2020 edition of Chinese Pharmacopoeia, these residual solvents in amitriptyline hydrochloride must be under to the following limits: toluene (%) $\leqslant 0.089\%$; isopropanol (%) $\leqslant 0.5\%$, tetrahydrofuran (%) $\leqslant 0.072\%$.

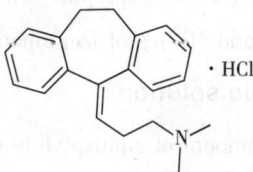

Fig. 4 – 1   The structure of amitriptyline hydrochloride

2. 2 The principle of temperature programming gas chromatography

For gas chromatography analysis of a mixture sample containing complicated components with widely differing boiling points and properties, if a lower column temperature is used, optimal separation and the appropriate retention are facilitated for the front peaks of elution, but the compounds with high boiling point will interact with the stationary phase for longer time, which leading to the long retention times and broaden peaks. If the column temperature is increased, all components will be accelerated and eluted from the column more quickly. Although the high boiling point compounds can obtain the appropriate retention and the good peak shape, the compounds with low boiling point will be eluted too fast. In the case of such problems, an optimal separation can often be achieved by temperature programming technology in gas chromatography.

Temperature programming means that the temperature of the chromatographic column increases either linearly or in steps manner at a preset rate during the running of the chromatography analysis, so that the compounds with different boiling points can be separated at the suitable temperature. Therefore, this technology ensures the good separation of low boiling point compounds and rapid elution of high boiling point compounds. Meanwhile, it also can accelerate the whole chromatographic separation process and achieves good peak shape. Because of the volatility and remarkably different boiling points of residual solvents, gas chromatography with temperature programming technology is commonly used to determine residual solvents in the drug substances.

3. Apparatus and Reagents

3. 1 Apparatus

Gas chromatography system; Flame ionization detector (FID); High purity nitrogen; Hydrogen; Air; Analytical balance; Microsyringe ($100\mu l$); Volume – tric flask (25ml, 100ml); Transfer pipettes (1ml, 2ml); Manual injection syringe for GC ($1\mu l$).

3. 2 Reagents

Amitriptyline hydrochloride (the purity $\geqslant 99\%$); Toluene, isopropanol and tetrahydrofuran are all analytical reagent (AR).

4. Experimental contents

4. 1 Preparation of the reference solution

Accurately weigh an appropriate amount of toluene, tetrahydrofuran and isopropanol, and then dissolve them with dimethyl formamide (DMF) to prepare a mixed solution containing about $17.8\mu g$ of toluene, $14.4\mu g$ of tetrahydrofuran and $100\mu g$ of isopropanol per 1ml.

4. 2 Preparation of the sample solution

Accurately weigh an appropriate amount of amitriptyline hydrochloride, dissolve in dimethyl formamide (DMF) to make a solution containing about 20mg amitriptyline hydrochloride per 1ml.

4. 3 Setting of gas chromatography conditions

Capillary column with 6% cyanopropyl phenyl – 94% dimethylpolysiloxane (30m × 0. 25mm ×

0.25μm)or a similar column is used as the stationary phase. The carrier gas is nitrogen. The column flow is about 4ml/min and the split ratio is 1 ∶ 20. The inlet temperature and hydrogen flame detector temperature are 160℃ and 250℃ ,respecttively. The column temperature is set according to the program:the column temperature starts at 80℃ and is maintained for 10minutes. The temperature is linearly increased at 20℃/min to 200℃ , and then the temperature is held at that value for 5minutes.

4. 4 The determination of residual solvent

Inject 1μl of the reference solution into the gas chromatography. The resolution between peaks each other should meet the requirements. Then inject 1μl of the sample solution and 1μl of the reference solution into the gas chromatography respectively to calculate the content of the residual toluene,tetrahydrofuran and isopropanol according to the peak areas by the external standard method. Their contents are all should meet the requirements in Chinese Pharmacopoeia.

5. Data record and processing

5. 1 Record for the preparation of the solutions

Table 4 – 1　Record for the preparation of the solutions

	Compound	Amount of the substance	Concentration of the solution
Reference solution	Tetrahydrofuran		
	Isopropanol		
	Toluene		
Sample solution	Amitriptyline hydrochloride		

5. 2 Original data for the determination of residual solvents

Table 4 – 2　Original data for the determination of residual solvents

		Reference solution			Sample solution		
		1	2	3	1	2	3
The peak area(A)	Tetrahydrofuran						
	Isopropanol						
	Toluene						
Resolution(R)	Tetrahydrofuran and isopropanol						
	Isopropanol and toluene						

Note:Boiling point:toluene:110. 6℃ ,isopropanol:82℃ , tetrahydrofuran:65. 4℃

5. 3 Calculation of the content of residual solvents

Calculate the concentration of each residual solvent in the sample solution according to the following equation:

$$Content(C_X) = (A_X/A_R) \cdot C_R.$$

Where,C_X is the concentration of the residual solvent in the sample solution;C_R is the concentration of the residual solvent in the reference solution;A_R is the peak area of the residual solvent in the reference solution;A_X is the peak area of the residual solvent in the sample solution.

The amount of each residual solvent in amitriptyline hydrochloride can be obtain according the percentage ratio between the concentration of residual solvents in the sample solution and the concentration of the sample solution (20mg/ml).

Table 4 – 3 The percentage of residual solvents in amitriptyline hydrochloride

	The percentage of residual solvents (%)		
	Tetrahydrofuran	Isopropanol	Toluene
1			
2			
3			
AVE			

6. Discussion and guidance

6. 1 Residual solvents and content limits

According to 2020 edition of Chinese Pharmacopoeia, the common residual solvents and their content limits are shown in the Table 4 – 4. Unless otherwise provision, the reside of the first, second and third types of solvents should conform to these limits. For other solvents, corresponding limits should be established according to the characteristics of production process to meet product specifications, the guide of the Good Manufacturing Practices (GMP) or other basic quality requirements. For new drug approval and registration, the residual solvents in drug substances are implemented in accordance with ICH requirements.

Table 4 – 4 The limits of common residual solvents in drug substances

Category I solvents (avoided use)		Category II solvents (restricted use)		Category III solvents (limited use by GMP or other quality requirements)		Category IV solvents (insufficient toxicological information)	
solvent name	limit (%)	solvent name	limit (%)	solvent name	limit (%)	solvent name	limit (%)
benzene	0.0002	acetonitrile	0.041	acetic acid	0.5	1,1 – diethoxy propane	
carbon tetrachloride	0.0004	chlorobenzene	0.036	acetone	0.5	1,1 – dimethoxy methane	
1,2 – dichloroethane	0.0005	trichloroethane	0.006	methoxy benzene	0.5	2,2 – dimethoxy propane	
1,1 – dichloroethylene	0.0008	cyclohexane	0.388	n – butyl alcohol	0.5	isooctane	
1,1,1 – trichloroethane	0.15	1,2 – dichloroethylene	0.187	s – butyl alcohol	0.5	isopropyl ether	
		dichloromethane	0.06	butyl acetate	0.5	methyl isopropyl ketone	
		1,2 – two methoxy ethane	0.01	t – butyl methyl ether	0.5	methyl tetrahydrofuran	
		N,N – dimethylacetamide	0.109	isopropyl benzene	0.5	petroleum ether	
		N,N – dimethylformamide	0.088	dimethyl sulfoxide	0.5	trichloroacetic acid	
		dioxane	0.038	ethanol	0.5	trifluoroacetic acid	
		2 – ethoxy ethanol	0.016	ethyl acetate	0.5		
		ethylene glycol	0.062	ether	0.5		
		formamide	0.022	ethyl formate	0.5		
		n – hexane	0.029	formic acid	0.5		
		methanol	0.300	n – heptane	0.5		

Category I solvents (avoided use)		Category II solvents (restricted use)		Category III solvents (limited use by GMP or other quality requirements)		Category IV solvents (insufficient toxicological information)	
solvent name	limit (%)	solvent name	limit (%)	solvent name	limit (%)	solvent name	limit (%)
		2 – methoxy ethanol	0.005	isobutyl acetate	0.5		
		methyl butyl ketone	0.005	isopropyl acetate	0.5		
		methyl cyclohexane	0.118	methyl acetate	0.5		
		N – methyl pyrrolidone	0.053	3 – methyl – 1 – butanol	0.5		
		nitromethane	0.005	butanone	0.5		
		pyridine	0.02	methyl isobutyl ketone	0.5		
		tetrahydrothiophene	0.016	isobutyl alcohol	0.5		
		tetrahydronaphthalene	0.01	n – pentane	0.5		
		tetrahydrofuran	0.072	n – amyl alcohol	0.5		
		toluene	0.089	n – propanol	0.5		
		1,1,2 – trichloroethylene	0.008	isopropanol	0.5		
		dimethylbenzene	0.217	propyl acetate	0.5		

6.2 The mode of temperature programming

Temperature programming method is a common and important technology in gas chromatography, whereby the column temperature is increased either continuously or in steps as the separation proceeds. For complex mixtures with a wide boiling range, it is often desirable to employ temperature programming to offer the optimal column temperature of each component in the sample. In practice, the first – order linearly or N – order linearly increasing temperature mode is widely used. In gas chromatography, the first – order linearly increasing temperature in can be used for samples with wide boiling point range and similar chemical properties (such as homologues); For the sample components with extremely different boiling point and the properties, N – order temperature program should be selected. The N should be based on the compromise between the number of compounds, the separation effect to be achieved, the conditions of the instrument and the nature of the components. During the process of programmed heating, it is necessary to wait for the chromatography to return to its initial state and stabilize after the completion of a temperature program before the next injection.

6.3 Sample injection methods for the determination of residual solvents.

Head – space injection is most commonly used for the determination of residual solvents. Since most residual solvents have low boiling points, it is convenient to analysis these volatile components in the vapor phase by heating the sample solution in the sealed head space bottle. According to the solubility of the sample and residual solvent, the appropriate solvent should be selected without interfering with the residual solvent in samples. For water – soluble drugs, water is usually used as the solvent. For non – water – soluble drugs, dimethyl formamide, dimethyl sulfoxide and other solvents with higher boiling point can be chosen. Headspace injection can eliminate or reduce the interference of drug matrix on the inlet and chromatographic separation, and has higher sensitivity than that of direct injection. Therefore, it has become the preferred method for the determination of residual solvents in drug substances. The disadvantage of this method is that operation should be equipped by the special head space injection device.

The direct injection method is mainly used for residual solvents with higher boiling point, such as dimethyl formamide, dimethyl sulfoxide, n – methyl pyrrolidone, etc. The sensitivity of direct injection method for such high boiling solvents is higher than that by head – space injection method. In the absence of head space injection device, direct injection method also can be used to determine the low boiling point solvent. It is should considered that the injection port is easily contaminated by drug matrix after multiple injection by direct injection.

第二章　药物高效液相色谱分析

Chapter 2　High Performance Liquid Chromatographic Analysis of Pharmaceuticals

实验五　高效液相色谱法基本技能实验

【实验目的】

1. 学习高效液相色谱仪的结构和工作原理。
2. 学习高效液相色谱法的操作流程。
3. 学习影响高效液相色谱分离效能的因素。

【实验原理】

1. 高效液相色谱色谱仪的结构和工作原理　采用高压输液泵将液体流动相泵入色谱柱，对样品进行分离测定的色谱方法称为高效液相色谱法（high performance liquid chromatography，HPLC）。高效液相色谱仪（HPLC）主要由输液系统（包括贮液瓶、脱气机和高压泵）、进样系统（包括进样器和进样阀）、分离系统（分离柱）、检

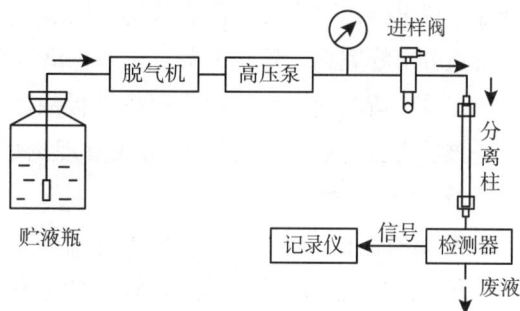

图 5-1　高效液相色谱仪的基本流程图

测系统（检测器）和数据处理系统（主机）组成（图 5-1）。流动相从贮液瓶中抽出，经过脱气机脱气后，由高压泵加压以恒定的流速流过进样阀，并进入色谱柱，最后到达检测器。样品在进样阀处注入，随流动相进入色谱柱进行色谱分离，被分离组分依次进入检测器产生信号，信号经色谱工作站采集、记录、处理后得到色谱图及分析报告。

2. 高效液相色谱影响色谱分离的因素

（1）固定相　固相种类是影响色谱分离效率的重要因素。一般根据相似相溶原则选择固定相。非极性键合相（C_{18}、C_8）广泛应用于非极性和中等极性样品分析。柱的填充质量也会对柱效产生影响，一般选用颗粒小且均匀的固定相，填充技术成熟的色谱柱。

（2）流动相　反相色谱的流动相通常以水作基础溶剂，再加入一定量的能与水互溶的极性调整剂，如甲醇、乙腈等。极性调整剂的性质及其所占比例对溶质的保留值和分离选择性有显著影响。

（3）柱温　柱温升高会使流动相黏度减小，从而加快分离过程，待测物的色谱保留减

弱。柱温降低则会使待测物保留增加，可能改善色谱峰之间的分离度。

（4）流速　流速根据色谱柱的粒径和内径选择最佳流速，以不超过高效液相色谱仪的使用压力为上限。流速的常规改变主要影响保留时间，流速越大，保留时间越短。根据检测器不同对峰面积也有不同影响，浓度型检测器的色谱峰响应与流速呈反比，质量型检测器的色谱峰不受流速影响。

【仪器与试剂】

1. 仪器　高效液相色谱仪，紫外检测器，色谱柱柱温箱，分析天平，量瓶（10ml、100ml），移液管（1ml、10ml），微量注射器（100μl）。

2. 试剂　苯、甲苯均为分析纯试剂，甲醇为色谱纯试剂，水为去离子水。

【实验内容】

1. 测试溶液的配制　分别配制50μg/ml苯的甲醇溶液、50μg/ml甲苯的甲醇溶液、50μg/ml苯和甲苯的混合甲醇溶液。

2. 色谱条件设置　色谱柱：Lichrospher ODS（250mm×4.6mm×5μm）或同类色谱柱；流动相：甲醇：水（80:20）（或根据优化结果选择）；流速1.0ml/min（或根据优化结果选择）；检测波长254nm；温度：室温（或根据优化结果选择）；进样量20μl。

3. 流动相比例的优化　选择不同的甲醇-水比例（80:20、75:25、70:30）考察流动相比例组成对色谱分离效能和柱压的影响。在同一流动相条件下，吸取20μl苯的甲醇溶液进样，待组分出峰完毕，停止采集，记录色谱峰保留时间；吸取20μl甲苯的甲醇溶液进样，待组分出峰完毕，停止采集，记录色谱峰保留时间；再吸取20μl的苯和甲苯的混合液进样，记录保留时间、峰面积、理论塔板数、分离度、对称因子，并重复进样3次考察重复性。该项实验主要考察流动相组成对理论塔板数、分离度、对称因子和重复性的影响，并选择最优的流动相条件。

4. 柱温的优化　在最优的流动相条件下，选择设定不同的柱温（45℃、40℃、35℃），按流动相比例优化的实验操作进行柱温的考察。该项实验主要考察柱温对保留时间、峰面积、理论塔板数、分离度、对称因子和重复性的影响，并选择最优柱温。

5. 流速的优化　在最优的流动相条件和柱温条件下，选择设定不同的流速（1.2ml/min、1.0ml/min、0.8ml/min），按流动相比例优化的实验操作进行流速考察。该项实验主要考察流速对保留时间、峰面积、理论塔板数、分离度、对称因子和重复性的影响，并选择最优流速。

【数据记录与处理】

1. 流动相比例优化数据记录

表5-1　流动相比例优化的数据记录

流动相比例	序号	色谱峰（苯） t_R（min）	色谱峰（甲苯） t_R（min）	苯和甲苯混合液								
				色谱峰（苯）				色谱峰（甲苯）				
				t_R（min）	A_1	n	T	t_R（min）	A_2	n	T	R	柱压
80:20	1												
	2												
	3												

续表

流动相比例	序号	色谱峰(苯) t_R(min)	色谱峰(甲苯) t_R(min)	苯和甲苯混合液 色谱峰(苯) t_R(min)	A_1	n	T	色谱峰(甲苯) t_R(min)	A_2	n	T	R	柱压
75:25	1												
	2												
	3												
70:30	1												
	2												
	3												

注：表中 t_R 为保留时间，A 为峰面积，n 为理论塔板数，T 为对称因子，R 为分离度。

2. 柱温优化数据记录

表5-2 柱温优化的数据记录

柱温(℃)	序号	色谱峰(苯) t_R(min)	色谱峰(甲苯) t_R(min)	苯和甲苯混合液 色谱峰(苯) t_R(min)	A_1	n	T	色谱峰(甲苯) t_R(min)	A_2	n	T	R	柱压
45	1												
	2												
	3												
40	1												
	2												
	3												
35	1												
	2												
	3												

注：表中 t_R 为保留时间，A 为峰面积，n 为理论塔板数，T 为对称因子，R 为分离度。

3. 流速优化数据记录

表5-3 流速优化的数据记录

流速(ml/min)	序号	色谱峰(苯) t_R(min)	色谱峰(甲苯) t_R(min)	苯和甲苯混合液 色谱峰(苯) t_R(min)	A_1	n	T	色谱峰(甲苯) t_R(min)	A_2	n	T	R	柱压
1.2	1												
	2												
	3												
1.0	1												
	2												
	3												

流速 （ml/min）	序号	色谱峰 （苯） t_R （min）	色谱峰 （甲苯） t_R （min）	苯和甲苯混合液									
				色谱峰 （苯）				色谱峰 （甲苯）					
				t_R （min）	A_1	n	T	t_R （min）	A_2	n	T	R	柱压
0.8	1												
	2												
	3												

注：表中 t_R 为保留时间，A 为峰面积，n 为理论塔板数，T 为对称因子，R 为分离度。

4. 流动相比例优化结果

表5-4　流动相比例优化结果

流动相比例		苯和甲苯混合液							
		苯			甲苯			苯和甲苯	
		A_1	n	T	A_2	n	T	R	A_1/A_2
80：20	平均值								
	$RSD\%$								
75：25	平均值								
	$RSD\%$								
70：30	平均值								
	$RSD\%$								

注：表中 $RSD\%$ 为相对标准偏差，A 为峰面积，n 为理论塔板数，T 为对称因子，R 为分离度。

5. 柱温优化结果

表5-5　柱温优化结果

柱温（℃）		苯和甲苯混合液							
		苯			甲苯			苯和甲苯	
		A_1	n	T	A_2	n	T	R	A_1/A_2
45	平均值								
	$RSD\%$								
40	平均值								
	$RSD\%$								
35	平均值								
	$RSD\%$								

注：表中 $RSD\%$ 为相对标准偏差，A 为峰面积，n 为理论塔板数，T 为对称因子，R 为分离度。

6. 流速优化结果

表5-6　流速优化结果

流速 （ml/min）		苯和甲苯混合液							
		苯			甲苯			苯和甲苯	
		A_1	n	T	A_2	n	T	R	A_1/A_2
1.2	平均值								
	$RSD\%$								

续表

流速 (ml/min)		苯和甲苯混合液								
		苯			甲苯			苯和甲苯	
		A_1	n	T	A_2	n	T	R	A_1/A_2
1.0	平均值								
	RSD%								
0.8	平均值								
	RSD%								

注：表中 RSD% 为相对标准偏差，A 为峰面积，n 为理论塔板数，T 为对称因子，R 为分离度。

【讨论与指导】

1. 高效液相色谱仪的基本操作方法

（1）开机　仪器操作前检查流动相贮液瓶中是否具有足够的流动相，吸液过滤器是否已插入储液瓶底部，废液瓶是否已倒空，所有排液管是否已妥善插在废液瓶中。确定无误后可开始操作。开启稳压电源后，依次打开输液泵、柱温箱、检测器和计算机电源。

（2）排气泡　将排液阀逆时针旋转180°至"Open"位置，按"Purge"键，观察输液泵中是否有气泡排出，确定管路中无气泡后，再按一次"Purge"键，使输液泵停止工作，再将排液阀顺时针旋转至"Close"位置，旋紧旋钮。

（3）设置参数　打开色谱工作站，连接仪器，打开高压输液泵，设定输液泵以低流速（0.2~0.5ml/min），开泵泵出流动相，在此条件下接色谱柱，接好后打开检测器，在参数设置目录下设定所需要的流速、检测波长等参数。

（4）进样与数据采集　检查设定的各项参数无误后，开始运行仪器，待各项参数均达到预设值时，在工作站下点击查看色谱基线，观察色谱基线是否平稳；待色谱基线稳定后，开始分析样品（如点击"单次分析"），进行样品信息的录入并保存；用进样针量取指定体积的试样，在流通阀"Load"状态下，插入进样针并注射样品到定量环（进样口），然后迅速旋转流通阀至"Inject"状态，连通定量环和色谱柱，即自动开始采样，观察出峰情况，直到所有组分出峰完毕，停止采集，保存色谱图文件。在离线工作站打开文件，调出所保存的色谱图和数据，进行数据处理。

（5）关机　试验结束后，需要对色谱系统进行冲洗，冲洗时可先关闭检测器电源。如果使用了含盐的流动相需要先用含10%甲醇的水冲洗系统20~30分钟，再更换流动相为纯甲醇冲洗色谱系统；如流动相不含盐可以直接用纯甲醇冲洗。冲洗完毕后，再依次关闭输液泵、柱温箱电源、控制电脑电源。如有必要卸下色谱柱，并及时按色谱柱说明书对色谱柱进行保养。

2. 高效液相色谱的注意事项

（1）流动相所采用的有机相需要色谱纯试剂级别，所使用的水为去离子水。

（2）有机相和水相两相混合后会产生较多气泡，如果采用两相混合的流动相需要采用低压脱气的方式，对于甲醇–水的两相混合流动相可以采用20分钟以上的超声脱气法。

（3）当排完气泡，停止"Purge"时，高压泵自动关闭，需重新打开泵，对流动相加压。

（4）安装色谱柱时，请注意柱管上标示的流动相流向，将色谱柱的入口端通过连接管与进样阀出口相连接；柱的出口与检测器连接。顺时针拧紧空心螺钉，直到拧不动为止，再用扳手继续顺时针拧1/4圈~1/2圈，切记不要用力过大。

（5）进样样品要求无微粒或可能阻死针头及进样阀的物质，样品溶液均要用0.45μm的滤膜过滤，防止微粒阻塞进样阀和减少对进样阀的磨损。

（6）手动进样时采用平头注射器吸取液体试样，应先用少量试样洗涤多次，再慢慢抽入试样，并且吸样量应为注射量的3~4倍。如内有气泡则将针头朝上，使气泡上升排出。

（7）六通进样阀进样前，旋转至"Load"位置，用平头注射器注入样品后，迅速转回至"Inject"位置进样。由于手柄处于"Load"和"Inject"之间时，流路中压力骤增，过高的压力会对柱头造成损坏，所以应尽快转动阀，不能停留在中途。

（8）在整个实验过程中，一定要留意观察泵的压力变化。确保在稳定的压力下进行实验。如压力几乎为"0"，可能泵没打开。如压力变小，可能出现了漏液。

（9）如实验过程中，不出现任何色谱峰信号，说明没有数据采集，可能主要跟检测器故障有关（如检测器线路松动、检测器设置错误、检测器电源未开或波长设定不准确）。

（10）为防止缓冲盐和其他残留物质留在进样系统中，每次实验结束后应冲洗进样器，通常用水和纯有机溶剂（如甲醇），在进样阀的"Load"和"Inject"位置反复冲洗。

Experiment 5　Basic Skill Experiment of High Performance Liquid Chromatography

1. Experimental purposes

1.1 To learn the structure and working principle of HPLC instrument.

1.2 To learn the operating procedures of HPLC method.

1.3 To learn factors affecting the separation efficiency of HPLC.

2. Experimental principles

2.1 The structure and working principle of HPLC instrument

High performance liquid chromatography (HPLC) is a chromatographic method for separation and determination of samples in which the liquid mobile phase is pumped into a column using a high pressure pump. HPLC is mainly composed of the mobilephase supply system including the solvents reservoirs, degassers and high pressure pumps, the sample injection system consisting of a sample injector and an injection valve, the separation system (chromatographic column), the detection system (detector) and the data processing system (Fig. 5 – 1). The mobile phase is extracted from the solvents reservoirs, degassed by degassing devices, pressurized by the high pressure pumps, flows through the injection valve at a constant flow rate, then enters the chromatographic column and finally reaches the detector orderly. Samples can be introduced manually into the injection valve with a syringe to fill the sample loop. After the injection, the samples are carried by the mobile phase that is forced under pressure into the chromatographic column for separation. The separated components enter the detector to generate signals, which are collected, recorded and processed by the chromatographic workstation to obtain chromatograms and analysis reports.

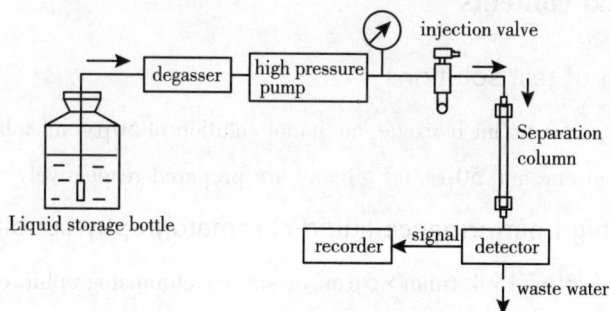

Fig. 5 - 1   The schematic diagram of a HPLC

2. 2 Factors affecting chromatographic separation by HPLC

a. Stationary phase   the type of solid phase is an important factor affecting the separation efficiency of chromatography. In general, the stationary phase is chosen according to the principles of similar compatibility and similar nature between the stationary phases and analytes. Nonpolar bonded phases (C_{18}, C_8) are widely used in the analysis of nonpolar and moderate polar samples. The filling of the column will also have an impact on the column efficiency. Generally, small and uniform stationary phases are selected to fill the column with mature technology.

b. Mobile phase   A mixture of water with one of the organic solvents which can be soluble in water is usually used in reversed phase chromatography. The organic solvents such as methanol, acetonitrile are added to adjust the polarity as modifier. The properties and content of the modifiers can significantly affect on the retention and separation selectivity of components.

c. Column temperature   The increase of column temperature will reduce the viscosity of mobile phase, thus accelerate the separation process and weaken the chromategraphic retention of the substance to be measured. On the contrary, the decrease of column temperature may improve the separations by increasing the retention of the components.

d. Flow rate   The best flow rate is chosen according to the size and inner diameter of the column and should not exceed the upper limit of the operating pressure of the HPLC. The flow rate mainly changes the retention time. For concentration sensitive detector, the chromatographic peak is inversely proportional to the flow rate. However, the chromatographic peak is not affected by the flow rate for the mass sensitive detector.

3. Apparatus and Reagents

3. 1 Apparatus

High performance liquid chromatography; Ultraviolet detector; Analytical balance; Volumetric flask (10ml,100ml);Transfer pipettes (1ml,10ml);Microsyringe (100μl).

3. 2 Reagents

Benzene and toluene are all analytical reagents (AR);Methanol is the reagent for chromatography;Water is deionized.

4. Experimental contents

4. 1 Preparation of test solutions

Methanol solution of 50μg/ml benzene,methanol solution of 50μg/ml toluene,mixed methanol solution of 50μg/ml benzene and 50μg/ml toluene are prepared respectively.

4. 2 Setting of high performance liquid chromatography conditions

Lichrospher ODS (250mm×4. 6mm×5μm) or similar chromatographic column is used as the stationary phase.

The mobile phase is a mixture of methanol and water (v/v = 80 : 20) or according to the optimized results and the flow rate is 1. 0ml/min or according to the optimized results.

The column temperature is room temperature or according to the optimized results.

The detection wavelength is 254nm and the injection volume is 20μl.

4. 3 Optimization of mobile phase ratios

Different ratios of methanol and water (80 : 20,75 : 25,70 : 30) are tested.

For each condition selected,inject 20μl of the methanol solution of benzene into HPLC system, after the elution of all components,stop acquirement and record the retention time of benzene;inject 20μl of the methanol solution of toluene into HPLC system,after the elution of all components,stop acquirement and record the retention time of toluene;inject 20μl of the mixed solution of benzene and toluene and record the retention times,peak areas,the number of theoretical plates,symmetry factors,resolution of benzene and toluene,and the reproducibility by repeating injection three times.

These experiments mainly are used to investigate the influence of the mobile phase on the number of theoretical plates,resolution,symmetry factors and reproducibilities. And then the optimal mobile phase ratio will be selected based on the above experimental results.

4. 4 Optimization of column temperature conditions

At the optimal mobile phase ratio,different column temperatures (45℃,40℃ and 35℃) are set for the optimization.

For each condition,the experimental procedures are the same as those in the optimization of mobile phase ratios.

These experiments mainly are used to investigate the influence of different column temperature on retention times,peak areas,the number of theoretical plates,resolution,symmetry factors and reproducibilities. And then the optimal column temperature can be selected.

4. 5 Optimization of flow rates

At the optimal mobile phase ratio and column temperature,three different flow rates of 1. 2ml/min,1ml/min and 0. 8ml/min are set for the optimization. At each flow rate,the experimental procedures are the same as those in the optimization of mobile phase ratios. These experiments mainly are used to investigate the influence of different flow rates on retention times, peak areas, the number of theoretical plates, resolution, symmetry factors and reproducibilities. And then the optimal flow rate can be selected.

5. Data record and processing

5. 1 The record for the optimization of mobile phase ratios

Table 5 – 1   The record for the optimization of mobile phase ratios

Mobile phase ratio		Benzene	Toluene	The mixed solution of benzene and toluene									
				Benzene				Toluene					
		t_R	t_R	t_R	A_1	n	T	t_R	A_2	n	T	R	Column pressure
80 : 20	1												
	2												
	3												
75 : 25	1												
	2												
	3												
70 : 30	1												
	2												
	3												

Note: t_R is retention time; A is peak area; n is the number of theoretical plates; T is symmetric factor; R is resolution.

5. 2 The record for the optimization of column temperature conditions

Table 5 – 2   The record for the optimization of column temperature conditions

Column temperature (℃)		Benzene	Toluene	The mixed solution of benzene and toluene									
				Benzene				Toluene					
		t_R	t_R	t_R	A_1	n	T	t_R	A_2	n	T	R	Column pressure
45	1												
	2												
	3												
40	1												
	2												
	3												
35	1												
	2												
	3												

Note: t_R is retention time; A is peak area; n is the number of theoretical plates; T is symmetric factor; R is resolution.

5. 3 The record for optimization of the flow rates

Table 5 – 3 The record for the optimization of flow rates

Flow rate (ml/min)	number	Benzene t_R	Toluene t_R	The mixed solution of benzene and toluene										
				Benzene				Toluene						
				t_R	A_1	n	T	t_R	A_2	n	T	R	Column pressure	
1. 2	1													
	2													
	3													
1. 0	1													
	2													
	3													
0. 8	1													
	2													
	3													

Note: t_R is retention time; A is peak area; n is the number of theoretical plates; T is symmetric factor; R is resolution.

5. 4 The results for the optimization of mobile phase ratios

Table 5 – 4 The results for the optimization of mobile phase ratios

Mobile phase ratio		The mixed solution of benzene and toluene							
		Benzene			Toluene				
		A_1	n	T	A_2	n	T	R	A_1/A_2
80 : 20	AVE								
	RSD%								
75 : 25	AVE								
	RSD%								
70 : 30	AVE								
	RSD%								

Note: $RSD\%$ is the relative standard deviation; A is peak area; n is the number of theoretical plates; T is the symmetric factor; R is resolution.

5. 5 The results for the optimization ofcolumn temperature conditions

Table 5 – 5 The results for the optimization of column temperature conditions

Column temperature (℃)		The mixed solution of benzene and toluene							
		Benzene			Toluene				
		A_1	n	T	A_2	n	T	R	A_1/A_2
45	AVE								
	RSD%								
40	AVE								
	RSD%								
35	AVE								
	RSD%								

Note: $RSD\%$ is the relative standard deviation; A is peak area; n is the number of theoretical plates; T is the symmetric factor; R is resolution (the separation degree).

5. 6 The results for the optimization of flow rates

Table 5 – 6   The results for the optimization of flow rates

Flow rate (ml/min)		The mixed solution of benzene and toluene							
		Benzene			Toluene				
		A_1	n	T	A_2	n	T	R	A_1/A_2
1. 2	AVE								
	RSD%								
1. 0	AVE								
	RSD%								
0. 8	AVE								
	RSD%								

Note: RSD% is the relative standard deviation; A is peak area; n is the number of theoretical plates; T is the symmetric factor; R is resolution.

6. Discussion and guidance

6. 1 Basic operation of HPLC

a. Starting up   Before the operation of the instrument, check whether there are enough mobile phases in the mobile phase reservoirs, whether the inlet filters have been immersed in the mobile phase, whether the waste liquid reservoir has been emptied, and whether all drain pipes have been properly inserted in the waste liquid reservoir. After confirmation, the next operation can be started. Turn on the powers of the stabilized voltage power supply, solvent supply module, column oven, detector, system controller and PC in turn.

b. Executing purge   Rotate the purge valve counter – clockwise 180 degrees to the "open" position, press the "purge" button, observe whether there are bubbles in the infusion pump to ensure there are no bubbles in the pipeline, and then press the "purge" button once again to stop the infusion pump, then rotate the purge valve back to the "close" position.

c. Setting parameters   Start the chromatographic workstation and connect the instruments. Start the high pressure pump and set a low flow rate in the range of 0. 2 ~ 0. 5ml/min to pump out the mobile phase, for the column connection. After the column connection, open the detector and set the flow rate, detection wavelength and other parameters under the parameter setting catalogue.

d. Injection and data acquisition   After setting parameters, start running the instrument in the workstation. Until all parameters are in ready, click "monitor" in method exercise to observe the chromatogram and ensure that the baseline of the detector as well as pump pressure is stable.

Start analysis of the samples (click "single analysis" button). First, input and save the sample information. Second, take a specified volume of sample with the microsyringe and inject it into the injection port. Third, observe the chromatogram until all components are eluted completely. Then stop the acquisition and save all data. Open the chromatogram in the offline workstation for the data processing.

e. Turning off   When analysis is completed, turn off the power of the detector and wash the chromatography system. If salt – containing mobile phase is used in the analysis, the system should be washed with water containing 10% methanol for 20 ~ 30minutes, and then the mobile phase is replaced by pure methanol for about 30minutes. If the mobile phase does not contain salt, it can be washed directly with pure methanol. After washing, turn off the powers of pump, the column temperature oven and PC. If necessary, remove the chromatographic column and maintain it in time according to the instructions of the column.

6. 2 Notes for the use of HPLC

a. The organic solvents used for HPLC should be HPLC grade reagents and the water should be deionized water.

b. Many bubbles will be generated when organic phases and water phases are mixed. Thus the mobile phase often need low – pressure degassing. The ultrasonic degassing method can be used for mobile phase of methanol – water for more than 20minutes.

c. When the purge is stopped, the high pressure pump is automatically closed, and the pump needs to be reopened.

d. When installing the chromatographic column, please pay attention to the flow direction of mobile phase indicated on the column tube. Connect the inlet end of the chromatographic column with the outlet of the injection valve by the connecting pipe. The exit of the column is connected to the detector. Tighten the hollow screw clockwise until it can't be moved, then continue to twist 1/4 to 1/2 turns clockwise with the wrench.

e. Some particles and contaminants in samples and mobile phases should be removed before analysis, so the sample solution and the mobile phase solution should be filtered through 0. 45μm filters to ptotect the pump and injection valve, and reduce contamination or plugging of the column.

f. The flat head syringe is usually used to take sample solutions 3 ~ 4 times of the size of sample loop during manual sample injection, and it should be washed for several times with a small amount of samples before its use. If there are bubbles in syringe, put the syringe upward to make the bubbles rise.

g. For the injection in the six – way valve, rotate the value to the position of "LOAD" and inject samples at "LOAD" status. Quickly return to the position of "INJECT" after sample injection. When the handle is in the halfway between "LOAD" and "INJECT", the flow pressure sharply increases and excessive pressure will damage the column head, so the valve should be rotated as soon as possible and cannot stay in the midway.

h. The pump pressure should be paid attention during the whole experiment process. Ensure that experiments are carried out under the stable pressure. If the pressure is almost "0", the pump may not be opened. If the pressure decreases, there might be a leakage.

i. If there is no chromatographic peak signal during the experiment, indicating no data collection, which mainly related to the failure of the detector (such as the loosening of the detector circuit, wrong detector setting, detector being not on or an inaccurate wavelength setting).

j. To prevent buffer salts and other residues from remaining in the injection system, the injector should be flushed repeatedly with water and pure organic solvents (such as methanol) at the "LOAD" and "INJECT" positions of the injection valve.

实验六　高效液相色谱法测定氯霉素及其制剂的含量

【实验目的】

1. 学习高效液相色谱法测定药物含量的流程。
2. 学习原料药和制剂含量的色谱测定方法。
3. 学习外标法和标准曲线法测定药物含量的原理。

【实验原理】

1. 氯霉素滴眼液　氯霉素（图 6 – 1）纯品是无色到白色或灰白色的针状或片状晶体或晶体粉末，易溶于甲醇，微溶于水。氯霉素分子中有 2 个不对称碳原子，所以氯霉素有 4 个光学异构体，其中只有左旋异构体具有抗菌能力。氯霉素的剂型包括片剂、胶囊、注射液、眼用软膏、滴眼液等。

氯霉素滴眼液常用于治疗沙眼、结膜炎、角膜炎、眼睑缘炎等。由于氯霉素干燥时稳定，但在溶液中高温、光照、强酸及碱性环境都会使氯霉素产生降解，因此氯霉素滴眼液在运输及储藏过程中需要遮光、密封、凉处（不超过 20℃）保存。

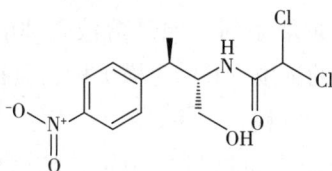

图 6 – 1　氯霉素的结构

2. 外标法与标准曲线法　外标法指取供试品溶液和对照品溶液，取一定量注入仪器，记录色谱图，测量对照品溶液和供试品溶液中待测组分的峰面积（或峰高），按下式计算含量：

$$含量(C_X) = C_R \times \frac{A_X}{A_R}$$

式中，A_R 为对照品溶液中待测物的峰面积（或峰高）；C_R 为对照品溶液中待测物的浓度；A_X 为供试品溶液中待测物的峰面积（或峰高）；C_X 为供试品溶液中待测物的浓度。

标准曲线法指配制一系列已知浓度的对照品溶液，在同一操作条件下注入色谱仪，测定其峰面积（或峰高），确定峰面积（峰高）与浓度的标准曲线，求出回归方程。

$$A = aC + b$$

式中，A 为待测组分峰面积（或峰高）；C 为待测组分浓度；a 为标准曲线斜率；b 为标准曲线截距。

然后在相同的条件下，精密量取供试品溶液，测定待测组分的峰面积（或峰高），根据回归方程，计算供试品中待测组分的浓度。

外标法是高效液相色谱法中最为常用的定量测定方法，在原料药和制剂的含量测定中均有广泛应用，但外标法的对照品溶液浓度与供试品溶液浓度应接近。相比于外标法，标

准曲线法更适用于待测物浓度范围较宽的测定。

【仪器与试剂】

1. 仪器 高效液相色谱仪，紫外检测器，分析天平，液相微量进样针（100μl），量瓶（10ml、50ml），移液管（5ml）。

2. 试剂 氯霉素滴眼液（市售品，12.5mg/5ml/支），氯霉素原料药（纯度＞99.0%），氯霉素对照品（中国食品药品检定研究院），甲醇为色谱级试剂，冰醋酸为分析纯，水为去离子水。

【实验内容】

1. 色谱条件的设置 色谱柱：Lichrospher ODS（250mm×4.6mm×5μm）或同类型色谱柱；流动相：甲醇－水－冰醋酸（65∶35∶0.1，v/v）（必要时可作调整）；柱温：室温；流速：1.0ml/min；进样量：20μl；检测波长：280nm；理论塔板数按氯霉素计算应不低于1800。

2. 系列对照品溶液的配制与测定 取氯霉素对照品约20mg，精密称定，置50ml量瓶中，加甲醇适量，振摇使溶解并稀释至刻度，摇匀，作为氯霉素对照品储备液。

精密量取储备液各1、2、3、4、5ml，分别置10ml量瓶中，加流动相稀释至刻度，摇匀，作为系列对照品溶液。精密量取系列对照品溶液各20μl，分别注入高效液相色谱仪，记录色谱图。以系列对照品溶液的浓度（C）为横坐标，氯霉素峰的峰面积（A）为纵坐标进行线性回归，得标准曲线和回归方程。

3. 原料药的含量测定 取氯霉素原料药约20mg，精密称定，置50ml量瓶中，加甲醇适量，振摇使溶解并稀释至刻度，摇匀，精密量取4ml，置10ml量瓶中，加流动相稀释至刻度，摇匀，作为原料药供试品溶液。精密量取原料药供试品溶液20μl，注入高效液相色谱仪，记录色谱图。按外标法以峰面积计算，即得氯霉素原料药的百分含量。同时将测得的氯霉素峰峰面积（A）代入回归方程，计算原料药供试品溶液中的氯霉素浓度，进一步计算氯霉素原料药的百分含量。

4. 氯霉素滴眼液的含量测定 精密量取氯霉素滴眼液2ml（约相当于氯霉素5mg），置50ml量瓶中，加流动相稀释至刻度，摇匀，作为氯霉素滴眼液供试品溶液。精密量取氯霉素滴眼液供试品溶液20μl，注入高效液相色谱仪，记录色谱图。按外标法以峰面积计算，即得氯霉素滴眼液的标示量百分含量。同时将测得的氯霉素峰峰面积（A）代入回归方程，计算氯霉素滴眼液供试品溶液中的氯霉素浓度，进一步计算氯霉素滴眼液的标示量百分含量。

【数据记录与处理】

1. 溶液的配制记录

表6－1 氯霉素对照品溶液的配制记录

对照品称样量 （mg）	对照品储备液浓度 （mg/ml）	系列对照品溶液浓度（mg/ml）				
		1	2	3	4	5

2. 回归方程的计算结果

表6-2 系列对照品溶液的回归方程计算结果

系列对照品溶液峰面积					回归方程	相关系数
1	2	3	4	5		

3. 含量测定结果

氯霉素原料药百分含量：含量 $= (C_X \times D) / m \times 100\%$。式中 C_X 为供试品溶液中氯霉素的浓度，D 为稀释倍数，m 为氯霉素原料药称样量。

表6-3 氯霉素原料药含量测定结果

	序号	称样量（mg）	峰面积	外标法计算结果（%）	标准曲线法计算结果（%）
原料药	1				
	2				
	3				

氯霉素滴眼液标示百分含量：含量 $= (C_X \times D) / S \times 100\%$。式中 C_X 为供试品溶液中氯霉素的浓度，D 为稀释倍数，S 为氯霉素滴眼液标示量。

表6-4 氯霉素滴眼液含量测定结果

	序号	取样量（ml）	峰面积	外标法计算结果（%）	标准曲线法计算结果（%）
氯霉素滴眼液	1				
	2				
	3				

【讨论与指导】

1. 药物的含量测定方法 药物的含量测定系指测定原料药或制剂中所含主成分的量，是药物质量控制的重要组成。药物的含量通常运用化学、物理学、生物学及微生物学的方法进行测定。《中国药典》（2020年版）正文各品种的含量测定以及附录所收载的用于药物含量、溶出或释放量测定的定量分析方法主要包括：容量分析法、光谱分析法和色谱分析法。其中，容量分析法、光谱法虽各有优势，但专属性均稍差；色谱法兼具分离和分析能力，可将各组分从混合物中分离后再选择性地对待测组分进行分析，该方法具有高灵敏度和高专属性，是分析混合物的最有力手段。色谱分析法除了在分离效能上更具优势外，还可根据色谱峰的峰面积或峰高对待测物的含量进行准确定量。

2. 原料药的含量测定结果表示方式 原料药的含量测定结果通常以百分含量（%）表示，公式如下：

$$百分含量（\%） = \frac{m_{测得量}}{m_{取样量}} \times 100\%$$

通常，首先以峰面积计，以外标/内标定量法求出待测物供试品溶液的浓度：

$$C_X = C_R \cdot A_X / A_R$$

式中，A_X 为供试品主成分的峰面积或峰高；C_X 为供试品的浓度；A_R 为对照品的峰面积；

C_R 为对照品的浓度。

若以内标法定量时，A_X 应乘上对应的校正因子 f 进行峰面积校正，然后计算得到供试品中 $m_{测得量}$，与 $m_{取样量}$ 进行对比，计算得到原料药的百分含量（%）。

3. 制剂的含量测定结果表示方式 药物制成制剂，均有其标示量，即每 1 个制剂单位所含有效成分的量。药物制剂的含量测定，均以其标示量为基础，检验制剂含量偏离标示量的程度，故制剂的含量测定结果以标示量的百分含量表示：

$$标示量百分含量（\%）= \frac{每个单位制剂的实际测得量}{标示量} \times 100\%$$

（1）对于片剂的含量测定，上述公式可进一步转换为：

$$标示量百分含量（\%）= \frac{（m_{测得量}/m_{取样量}）\times 平均片重}{标示量} \times 100\%$$

（2）对于注射液等液体制剂的含量测定，公式为：

$$标示量百分含量（\%）= \frac{C_{实测}}{C_{标示}} \times 100\%$$

4. 药物的稳定性 药品的稳定性特指其保持理化性质和生物学特性不变的能力。药品的稳定性与药物在临床应用过程中的疗效与安全性有着密不可分的关系，若药品的稳定性差，发生降解而引起质量变化，则不仅有可能使药效降低，而且生成的杂质还有可能产生毒副作用，因此需要考察稳定性试验。

稳定性试验的目的是提供原料药或制剂在各种环境因素如温度、湿度和光等条件影响下，其质量随时间变化的情况，并且由此建立原料药的再试验期或制剂的货架期以及推荐的贮存条件。

Experiment 6　Assay of Chloramphenicol and its Preparation by High Performance Liquid Chromatography

1. Experimental purposes

1. 1 To learn the procedures for the assay by high performance liquid chromatography.

1. 2 To learn the chromatographic method for the assay of active pharmaceutical ingredients and pharmaceutical preparations.

1. 3 To learn the principle for the assay by the external standard method and the calibration curve method.

2. Experimental principles

2. 1 The chloramphenicol ophthalmic solution

Chloramphenicol（Fig. 6 – 1）appears as colorless to white or greyish white, acicular or flaky crystals or crystalline powder, which is freely soluble in methanol and slightly soluble in water. Chloramphenicol contains two asymmetric carbon atoms in the molecule, thus four optical isomers of chloramphenicol exist, of which only the levorotatory isomer has antibacterial activity. The dosage forms of chloramphenicol include tablets, capsules, injections, ophthalmic ointment, ophthalmic solutions, etc.

The chloramphenicol ophthalmic solution is commonly used to treat trachoma, conjunctivitis, keratitis, blepharitis, etc. Dried chloramphenicol is stable, but it will degrade under high temperature, light, strongly acidic or alkaline environment in solution. Therefore, the chloramphenicol ophthalmic solution needs to be light – shielded, sealed and cool (no more than 20℃) during transportation and storage.

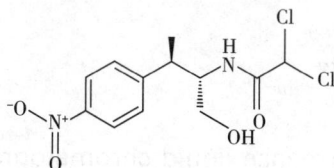

Fig. 6 – 1   The structure of chloramphenicol

2. 2 The external standard method and the calibration curve method

The external standard method means that the sample solution and the reference solution are injected into the chromatography system. The peak area or peak height of the analyte is measured to calculate the content as follows:

$$Content(C_X) = C_R \times \frac{A_X}{A_R}$$

Where, A_R is the peak area or peak height of analyte in the reference solution; C_R is the concentration of analyte in the reference solution; A_X is the peak area or peak height of analyte in the sample solution; C_X is the concentration of analyte in the sample solution.

The calibration curve method means a series of reference solutions is prepared and injected into the chromatography system. Then the peak areas (or peak heights) of analyte in the reference solutions are plotted versus the corresponding concentrations to get the regression equation as follows:

$$A = aC + b$$

Where, A is the peak area or peak height of analyte; C is the concentration of analyte; a is the slope of calibration curve; b is the intercept of calibration curve.

Then the sample solution is injected into the chromatography system under the same operating conditions. The peak areas or peak heights of analyte in the sample solution is used to calculate the concentration of analyte in sample solution according to the regression equation.

The external standard method is the most commonly used quantitative method in high performance liquid chromatography. It is widely applied in the assay of active pharmaceutical ingredients and pharmaceutical preparations. Compared with the external standard method, the calibration curve method is more suitable for the determination of samples with a wide concentration range.

3. Apparatus and Reagents

3. 1 Apparatus

High performance liquid chromatography; Ultraviolet detector; Analytical balance; Manual injection syringe for HPLC (100μl); Volumetric flask (10ml,50ml); Transfer pipettes (5ml).

3. 2 Reagents

Chloramphenicol ophthalmic solution (commercial products, 12. 5mg / 5ml / unit); Chloramphenicol (purity is more than 99. 0%); Chloramphenicol reference substance (National institute for the control of pharmaceutical and biological products); Methanol is the HPLC grade reagent and glacial acetic acid is analytical reagent (AR); Water is deionized.

4. Experimental contents

4. 1 Setting of high performance liquid chromatography conditions

Lichrospher ODS (250mm × 4. 6mm × 5μm) or similar chromatographic column is used as the stationary phase. The mobile phase is methanol:water:glacial acetic acid (65 : 35 : 0. 1,v/v) and the flow rate is 1. 0ml/min. The column temperature is room temperature. The detection wavelength is 280nm and the inject volume is 20μl. The number of theoretical plates should not be less than 1800 according to the peak of chloramphenicol.

4. 2 Preparation and determination of a series of reference solutions

Accurately weigh 20mg of chloramphenicol reference substance to a 50ml volumetric flask, then dissolve and dilute it with methanol to the mark and shake well as the stock solution.

Accurately pipette 1,2,3,4 and 5ml of the stock solution to five 10ml volumetric flasks respectively, then dilute them with mobile phase to the mark and shake well as a series of reference solutions. Inject 20μl of the above solutions into the high performance liquid chromatography system and record the chromatograms. The calibration curves and the regression equation are obtained by plotting the peak areas versus the corresponding concentrations.

4. 3 Assay of chloramphenicol

Accurately weigh 20mg of chloramphenicol to a 50ml volumetric flask, then dissolve and dilute it with methanol to the mark and shake well. Accurately pipette 4ml of the solution to a 10ml volumetric flask, then dilute it with the mobile phase to the mark and shake well. Inject 20μl of the above solution into the high performance liquid chromatography system and record the chromatograms. The obtained peak area of chloramphenicol is used to calculate the percentage content of chloramphenicol by the external standard method and the calibration curve method.

4. 4 Assay of chloramphenicol ophthalmic solution

Accurately pipette 2ml of chloramphenicol ophthalmic solution (equivalent to about 5mg of chloramphenicol) to a 10ml volumetric flask, then dilute it with the mobile phase to the mark and shake well. Inject 20μl of the above solution into the high performance liquid chromatography system and record the chromatograms. The obtained peak area of chloramphenicol is used to calculate the percentage of labelled amount in chloramphenicol ophthalmic solution by the external standard method and the calibration curve method.

5. Data record and processing

5. 1 Record for the preparation of the reference solutions

Table 6 – 1　Record for the preparation of the reference solutions

Amount of reference substance(mg)	Concentration of the stock solution(mg/ml)	Concentration of a series of reference solution(mg/ml)				
		1	2	3	4	5

5. 2 Calculation results of regression equation

Table 6 – 2　The original data and calculation results of regression equation

Peak area of reference solutions					Regression equation	Correlation coefficient
1	2	3	4	5		

5. 3 Assay results

The percentage content of chloramphenicol is calculated as follows: Content $(\%) = (C_X \times D)/m \times 100\%$. Where, C_X is the concentration of chloramphenicol in the sample solution; D is the dilute multiple during the preparation of the sample solution; m is the amount of chloramphenicol.

Table 6 – 3　The results for assay of chloramphenicol

	Number	Sample weight(mg)	Peak area	Results by the external standard method	Results by the calibration curve method
Chloramphenicol substance	1				
	2				
	3				

The percentage of labelled amount of chloramphenicol in thechloramphenicol ophthalmic solution is calculated as follows: Content $(\%) = (C_X \times D)/S \times 100\%$. Where: C_X is the concentration of chloramphenicol in the sample solution; D is the dilute multiple during the preparation of the sample solution; S is the labelled amount (mg/ml).

Table 6 – 4　The results for assay of chloramphenicol ophthalmic solutions

	Number	Sample volume(ml)	Peak area	Results by the external standard method	Results by the calibration curve method
Chloramphenicol ophthalmic solution	1				
	2				
	3				

6. Discussion and guidance

6. 1 Method for the assay

The assay means the determination the content of principal ingredient in active pharmaceutical ingredients or pharmaceutical preparations, which is very important for the quality control of drugs. The assay method includes these techniques in chemistry, physics, biology and microbiology. The assay methods in the text and the appendix of Pharmacopoeia of the People's Republic of China for the determination of the drug content, dissolution or release include the volumetric method, the spectroscopic method and the chromatographic method. Although the volumetric method and the spectroscopic method have some advantages, the specificity of these two methods is poor. Compared with them, the chromatographic method has the ability to separate and analyze simultaneously. The components can be separated from the mixture and then analyzed selectively. Therefore, the chromatographic method is the most powerful technique to analyze mixtures, which has high sensitivity and specificity. In addition to the advantages of separation efficiency, the chromatographic method can also accurately quantify the content of the measured substance according to the peak area or peak height of the chromatographic peak.

6. 2 Expression of the content results of active pharmaceutical ingredients

The content determination results of active pharmaceutical ingredients are usually expressed in the percentage content (%) and the formula is as follows:

$$\text{The percentage content}(\%) = \frac{m_{\text{Determination}}}{m_{\text{Sampling}}} \times 100\%$$

In general, the concentration of the sample solution is calculated by the external/internal standard method based on the peak area:

$$C_X = C_R \cdot A_X / A_R$$

Where, A_R is the peak area or peak height of analyte in standard solution; C_R is the concentration of the standard solution; A_X is the peak area or peak height of analyte in sample solution; C_X is the concentration of the sample solution.

When quantifying by internal standard method, A_X should be multiplied by the correction factor f to correct the peak area. Then $m_{\text{Determination}}$ in the samples is calculated and compared with m_{Sampling} to get the percentage content (%) of substance.

6. 3 Expression of the content results of pharmaceutical preparations

Each pharmaceutical preparation has its labelled amount, that is the quantity of active ingredients contained in each preparation unit.

The determination of the content of pharmaceutical preparations is based on the labelled amount to inspect the degree that the content deviates from the labelled amount. The content determination results of pharmaceutical preparations are usually expressed in the percentage of labelled amount (%), and the formula is as follows:

$$\text{The percentage of labelled amount}(\%) = \frac{\text{The actual measured quantity in each preparation unit}}{\text{labelled amount}} \times 100\%$$

(1) For the determination of tablet content, the above formula can be further converted into:

$$\text{The percentage of labelled amount}(\%) = \frac{\left(\dfrac{m_{\text{Determination}}}{m_{\text{Sampling}}} \times \text{The percentage weight of tablet}\right)}{\text{labelled amount}} \times 100\%$$

(2) For the determination of liquid preparations such as injections, the formula is:

$$\text{The percentage of labelled amount}(\%) = \frac{c_{\text{Determination}}}{c_{\text{labelledamount}}} \times 100\%$$

6.4 Drug stability

Drug stability refers to the ability to maintain its physical and chemical properties and biological characteristics. Drug stability is closely related to the efficacy and safety of drugs in the process of clinical application. If the stability of drugs is poor, degradation will occur and cause quality changes, which is not only possible to reduce the efficacy, but also the generated impurities may produce toxicities. Therefore, it is necessary to investigate the stability of drugs.

The purpose of stability testing is to provide evidences on how the quality of substance or preparations change varies with time under the influence of a variety of environmental factors such as temperature, humidity light, and to establish a retest period for the substance or a shelf life for preparations and recommended storage conditions.

实验七　HPLC 法测定阿司匹林中水杨酸杂质

【实验目的】

1. 学习色谱法定量测定药物中杂质的方法。
2. 学习高效液相色谱中紫外检测器的原理。
3. 学习系统适用性试验的意义。

扫码"学一学"

【实验原理】

1. 阿司匹林与水杨酸　阿司匹林，又称为 2 -（乙酰氧基）苯甲酸，具有解热镇痛和消炎作用，临床上亦可用作抗血栓药物。其常规合成方法（图 7 - 1）是以水杨酸与乙酸酐为反应原料，在浓硫酸催化下，使水杨酸的羟基被乙酰化而得到，通过重结晶方法进行纯化。水杨酸既是阿司匹林的合成原料，也可能是阿司匹林在储存过程中酯键水解后生成的降解产物。因此需要对阿司匹林中的水杨酸杂质进行控制。

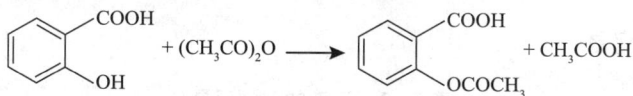

图 7 - 1　阿司匹林的合成方法

2. 紫外检测器原理　紫外检测器（ultraviolet absorption detector，UVD）是高效液相色谱仪中使用最广泛的一种检测器。紫外检测器是通过测定样品在检测池中吸收紫外 - 可见光的大小来确定样品含量的。根据朗伯 - 比尔定律，当一束单色光辐射通过物质的稀溶液时，如果溶剂不吸收光，则溶液的吸光度与吸光物质的浓度和光经过的溶液的距离成正比。

$$A = \varepsilon b c \qquad\qquad (7-1)$$

式中，A 为吸光度（absorbance）；又称光密度（optical density，OD）或消光值（extinction，E）；b 为光在溶液中经过的距离，一般为吸收池厚度；c 是吸光物质溶液的浓度；

ε 为吸光系数。

由上式可见，吸光度与吸光系数、溶液浓度和光路长度成线性关系，当紫外检测器检测样品的光路长度一定时，ε 值越大，灵敏度越高。而 ε 的数值大小取决于波长和样品物质的性质，它表明物质分子对特定波长的吸收能力。

【仪器与试剂】

1. 仪器 高效液相色谱仪，紫外检测器，分析天平，液相微量进样针（100μl），量瓶（10ml、100ml），移液管（5ml）。

2. 试剂 水杨酸对照品（中国食品药品检定研究院），阿司匹林供试品（市售），冰醋酸为分析纯试剂，甲醇为色谱级试剂，水为去离子水。

【实验内容】

1. 对照品溶液的配制 取水杨酸对照品约20mg，精密称定，置100ml量瓶中，加1%冰醋酸的甲醇溶液适量使溶解并稀释至刻度，摇匀，精密量取5ml，置100ml量瓶中，用1%冰醋酸的甲醇溶液稀释至刻度，摇匀，作为水杨酸对照品溶液（10μg/ml）。

2. 供试品溶液的配制 取阿司匹林供试品约0.1g，精密称定，置10ml量瓶中，加1%冰醋酸的甲醇溶液适量，振摇使溶解，并稀释至刻度，摇匀，作为阿司匹林供试品溶液（10mg/ml）。

3. 色谱条件的设置 色谱柱：Lichrospher ODS（250mm×4.6mm×5μm）或同类型色谱柱；流动相：甲醇-水-冰醋酸（70:30:0.1）（必要时可作调整）；温度：室温；流速：1.0ml/min；进样量：20μl；检测波长：276nm、303nm。

4. 游离水杨酸的测定 立即精密量取水杨酸对照品溶液和阿司匹林供试品溶液各20μl，分别注入液相色谱仪，记录色谱图。调整流动相条件，使理论板数按水杨酸峰计算不低于5000，阿司匹林峰与水杨酸峰的分离度应符合要求。供试品溶液色谱图中如果有与水杨酸峰保留时间一致的色谱峰，按外标法以峰面积计算，不得过0.1%。

【数据记录与处理】

1. 溶液的配制记录

表7-1 溶液的配制记录

对照品的称样量	对照品溶液浓度（C_R）	供试品的称样量	供试品的浓度（C_S）

2. 系统适用性实验结果

表7-2 适用性实验结果

样品	保留时间	理论塔板数	对称因子	分离度
水杨酸对照品溶液				
阿司匹林供试溶液				

3. 游离水杨酸的测定结果 根据外标法计算阿司匹林供试品溶液中水杨酸浓度 $C_X = A_X / (A_R / C_R)$，式中，A_X 为阿司匹林供试品溶液中水杨酸峰面积，A_R 为水杨酸峰对照品溶液中水杨酸峰面积，C_R 为水杨酸峰对照品溶液的浓度。

进而计算阿司匹林中游离水杨酸的含量（%）= $C_X / C_S \times 100\%$，式中 C_S 为阿司匹林供试品溶液的浓度。

表 7-3 游离水杨酸的测定结果

		峰面积（A_{276}）	峰面积（A_{303}）
水杨酸对照品	1		
	2		
	3		
阿司匹林供试品	1		
	2		
	3		
游离水杨酸的含量	平均值		

【实验指导与讨论】

1. 药物中的杂质控制 在药物的生产和贮藏过程中，常常会将一些杂质引入到药物中而使药物的纯度受到影响。这些杂质既无治疗作用，还可能影响药物的稳定性和疗效，甚至损害人们的健康，因此，必须对药物中的杂质进行检查，以保证药品质量和临床用药安全有效。

有关物质是药物中的一类特殊杂质，是指与药物主成分的结构母核类似或者具有渊源关系的杂质统称，一般包括药物生产和贮藏过程中可能引入的起始原料、中间体、反应副产物和降解产物等杂质。药物中有关物质的测定目前主要采用高效液相色谱法，即利用高效液相色谱法分离药物与其有关物质，进而对有关物质进行控制。由于色谱法可以通过峰面积进行杂质定量，因此根据定量方式的不同，可以分为杂质对照品法、主成分自身对照法、加校正因子的主成分自身对照法和面积归一化法。

2. 药物中杂质的定量测定方法

（1）杂质对照品法 方法：杂质测定时，配制杂质对照品溶液和供试品溶液，分别取一定量注入色谱仪，测定杂质对照品溶液和供试品溶液中杂质峰的响应，按外标法（必要时采用内标法）计算杂质的浓度。

该法定量比较准确，但由于每次测定时必须使用杂质对照品，因此杂质对照品用量极大，仅适用于杂质对照品容易大量获取的情况。

（2）加校正因子的主成分自身对照法 方法：在测定方法建立时，配制杂质对照品溶液和药物对照品溶液，得到杂质相对于主成分的相对保留时间和校正因子（f）。校正因子计算公式如下：

$$f = \frac{A_S / C_S}{A_R / C_R}$$

式中，A_S 为药物对照品的峰面积；A_R 为杂质对照品的峰面积；C_S 为药物对照品的浓度；C_R 为杂质对照品的浓度。

杂质测定时，以药物对照品溶液或供试品溶液的稀释液作为杂质对照溶液，通过测定供试品溶液中杂质峰的响应，乘以相应的校正因子后，与对照溶液中主成分的峰面积比较，计算杂质含量。

$$C_X = \frac{A_X}{A_S'/C_S'} \cdot f$$

式中，A_X 为供试品溶液杂质的峰面积；A_S' 为对照溶液药物主成分的峰面积；C_X 为杂质的浓度；C_S' 为对照溶液中药物的浓度。

本法的优点是仅在方法建立过程中需要杂质对照品，通过以主成分为参照，用相对保留时间定位、校正因子用于校正该杂质的实测峰面积。方法载入质量标准后，在日常检验中可以根据方法所规定的相对保留时间和校正因子测定药物中的杂质含量，无需再使用杂质对照品。但当校正因子测定值 ≤ 0.2 或 ≥ 5 时，为减少测定误差，应改用杂质对照品法。

（3）不加校正因子的主成分自身对照法　方法：杂质测定时，以药物对照品溶液或供试品溶液的稀释液为杂质对照溶液，通过测定供试品溶液中杂质峰的响应，与对照溶液中主成分的峰面积比较，按外标法计算杂质含量。

该法仅当杂质与主成分的校正因子在0.9～1.1范围内时适用，超过0.9～1.1范围内，应加入校正因子。但对于未知结构杂质或无法得到对照品的杂质，该法为一种权宜之计，如通过该法测得杂质含量较高（≥ 0.2%），应鉴定杂质结构、获取杂质对照品并测定其与主成分之间的校正因子。

（4）面积归一化法　方法：取供试品溶液适量，注入液相色谱仪，记录色谱图。测量各峰的面积和色谱图中除溶剂峰以外的总色谱峰面积，计算各杂质峰面积占总峰面积的百分率，应不得超过限量。

虽然该法的原理较为简单，测定过程也似乎更为简洁，但是《中国药典》（2020年版）对本法的使用作了明确的限定：除另有规定外，一般不宜用于微量杂质的检查。除杂质与药物之间的峰响应差别可能较大外，主要原因是药物中的杂质含量与主成分的含量相差悬殊，峰面积与浓度之间的线性关系往往会发生偏差，相比于主成分自身对照法，面积归一化法会产生更大的测定误差。因此，该方法通常只适用于药物中限度范围较宽的杂质测定。

3. 系统适用性　色谱分析方法在使用时，每次在分析样品前，操作人员必须确认色谱系统和操作步骤来保证数据的准确性，这就要依靠系统适用性试验（system suitability test）来完成。系统适应性实验即用规定的对照品对仪器进行试验和调整，应达到规定的要求；或规定分析状态下色谱柱的最小理论塔板数、分离度、重复性和拖尾因子。

Experiment 7　Determination of Salicylic Acid Impurity in Aspirin by HPLC

1. Experimental purposes

1.1 To learn the chromatographic method for the quantitative determination of impurities.

1. 2 To learn the principle of ultraviolet detector in HPLC.

1. 3 To learn the necessary of system suitability for the chromatographic separation.

2. Experimental principles

2. 1 Introduction of aspirin and salicylic acid

Aspirin, known as 2 – (acetyloxy) benzoic acid, has antipyretic, analgesic and anti – inflammatory effects. It is also used as an antithrombotic drug in clinic. The acetylation of salicylic acid with acetic anhydride under the catalysis of concentrated sulfuric acid is a conventional synthesis method of aspirin (Fig. 7 – 1). Then the synthesis product is further purified by re – crystallization to obtain the final product as the active pharmaceutical ingredient. Therefore, salicylic acid is the important impurity as the raw material during the synthesis of aspirin. Otherwise, salicylic acid is also the degradation (the ester bond hydrolysis) product of aspirin during the storage procedures. Therefore, it is extreme important to control the content of salicylic acid impurity in aspirin.

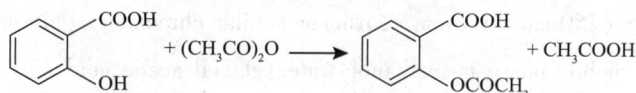

Fig. 7 – 1   The synthesis method of aspirin

2. 2 The principle of ultraviolet detector

Ultraviolet absorption detector is one of the most widely used detectors in HPLC. UV detector determines the sample content by measuring the absorbance of the UV – visible light in the detection cell. According to Lambert – Bill's law, when a beam of monochromatic light passes through a dilute solution, if the solvent does not absorb light, the absorbance of the solution is proportional to the concentration of the absorbent substance and the distance from the solution through which the light passes.

$$A = \varepsilon bc \qquad\qquad (7-1)$$

Where, A is the absorbance, also named as optical density (OD) or extinction (E); b is the distance that the light passes through the solution, usually is the thickness of the absorption cell; c is the concentration of the absorbent substance solution; ε is the absorption coefficient.

It can be seen from the above equation, the absorbance is in a straight line with the absorption coefficient, the solution concentration and the length of the light path. When the distance of the light is fixed, the larger the ε value, the higher the sensitivity of a UV detector. The ε value depends on the wavelength and the nature of the sample, which indicates the absorption capacity of molecules at a particular wavelength.

3. Apparatus and Reagents

3. 1 Apparatus

High performance liquid chromatography; Ultraviolet detector; Analytical balance; Volumetric flask (10ml, 100ml); Pipettes (5ml); Manual syringe for LC (100μl).

3. 2 Reagents

Salicylic acid reference substance (National Institute for the Control of Pharmaceutical and Biological Products); Aspirin (commercially available); Glacial acetic acid is analytical reagent (AR). Acetonitrile and methanol are reagents for HPLC; Water is the ultra – pure water.

4. Experimental contents

4. 1 Preparation of the reference solution

Accurately weigh 20mg salicylic acid reference substance to a 100ml volumetric flask, then dissolve and dilute it with the methanol solution containing 1% glacial acetic acid to the mark and shake well as the stock solution. Transfer 5ml solution into a 100ml volumetric flask, then dilute with the methanol solution containing 1% glacial acetic acid as the reference solution (10μg/ml).

4. 2 Preparation of the sample solution

Accurately weigh 0. 1g aspirin to a 10ml volumetric flask, then dissolve and dilute it with the methanol solution containing 1% glacial acetic acid to the mark and shake well as the sample solution.

4. 3 Setting of high performance liquid chromatography conditions

Lichrospher ODS (250mm × 4. 6mm × 5μm) or similar chromatographic column is used as the stationary phase. The mobile phase is methanol: water: glacial acetic acid (70 : 30 : 0. 1, v/v) and the flow rate is 1. 0ml/min. The column temperature is room temperature. The detection wavelength is 276nm and 303nm. The inject volume is 20μl.

4. 4 Determination of free salicylic acid

After the preparation of the reference solution and the sample solution, immediately inject 10μl of each solution into the high performance liquid chromategraphy system and record the chromatograms, respectively. Adjust the mobile phase condition to ensure that the theoretical plate number of salicylic acid peak is no less than 5000 and the resolution between aspirin and salicylic acid is no less than 1. 5. The salicylic acid impurity in the sample solution should be less than 0. 1% by the external standard method.

5. Data record and processing

5. 1 Record for the preparation of the solutions

Table 7 – 1   Record for the preparation of the solutions

Amount of reference substance (mg)	Concentration of the reference solution (C_R)	Amount of sample (mg)	Concentration of the sample solution (C_S)

5. 2 System suitability test

Table 7 – 2   System suitability test

Sample	Retention time(min)	Theoretical plate number	Symmetry factor	Resolution factor
Salicylic acid reference solution				
Aspirin test solution				

5. 3 Determination of free salicylic acid

The concentration of salicylic acid in the sample solution is calculated as follows: $C_X = A_X/(A_R/C_R)$. Where, C_X is the concentration of salicylic acid in the sample solution; C_R is the concentration of salicylic acid in the reference solution; A_X is the peak area of salicylic acid in the sample solution; A_R is the peak area of salicylic acid in the reference solution.

Then the content of salicylic acid in the sample solution can be obtained as follows: Content (%) $= C_X/C_S \times 100\%$. Where: C_X is the concentration of salicylic acid in the sample solution; C_S is the concentration of aspirin in the sample solution.

Table 7 − 3 The content of salicylic acid in aspirin

Sample	Number of injection	Peak area (A_{276})	Peak area (A_{303})
Then reference solution	1		
	2		
	3		
The sample solution	1		
	2		
	3		
The content of salicylic acid in aspirin	Ave		

6. Discussion and guidance

6. 1 The control of impurities in drugs

During the production and storage procedures of drugs, various impurities are often introduced into the drugs, resulting to the decrease of the drug purity. These impurities have no therapeutic effect, or affect the stability and efficacy of drugs, and even damage the health of people. Therefore, it is necessary to control these impurities to ensure the quality of drugs and the safety or efficacy of clinical medication.

Related substances are a kind of special impurities in drugs with similar structures or related to the principle components of drugs. These impurities may come from the raw materials, intermediates, by − products and degradation of the substance during the production and storage period. At present, high performance liquid chromatography (HPLC) is a powerful tool for the separation and determination of the related substances in drugs. The control methods of impurity in drugs by the chromatographic peak area include: reference substance method, main component self − control method with the corrected factor, main component self − control method without the corrected factor and peak area normalization method.

6. 2 The quantitative methods for the determination of impurities in drugs

a. Reference substance method   Method: During the determination of a known impurity, the impurity reference solution and the sample solution are prepared and injected into the chromatography system to obtain the peak responses of impurity in each solution. Then the concentration of impurity can be calculated by the external standard method.

This method is more accurate than any other methods, but the disadvantage of the reference substance method is the need of the impurity reference substance for the each analysis. Therefore, this method is suitable for the control of these cheap known impurities.

b. Main component self – control method with the corrected factor　Method: During the development of the impurity control method, the impurity reference solution and the drug reference substance solution are prepared and injected into the chromatography system to obtain the peak responses of impurity in each solution to obtain the correction factor (f) between the drug and impurity. The correction factor (f) of each known impurity is calculated as follows:

$$f = \frac{A_S/C_S}{A_R/C_R}$$

Where, A_S is the peak area of drug reference substance; A_R is the peak area of impurity reference substance; C_S is the concentration of drug reference substance; C_R is the concentration of impurity reference substance.

Then during the determination of this known impurity, the drug reference substance solution or the diluted sample solution is used as the impurity reference solution. Measure the peak area of this impurity in the sample solution and the peak area of the principal component in the reference solution. The concentration of impurity in the sample solution can be calculated as follows:

$$C_X = \frac{A_X}{A_S'/C_S'} \cdot f$$

Where, A_X is the peak area of the impurity in sample solution; A_S' is the peak area of the principal component in the reference solution; C_X is the concentration of the impurity in the sample solution; C_S' is the concentration of the principal component in the reference solution.

The advantage of this method is the no need of the impurity reference standard for each analysis. By using the principle component as the control, the correction factor and the relative retention time of impurity are obtained during the development of the impurity control method. Because the correction factor and relative retention time of impurities are recorded in the quality specification of drug, it is very convenient to use the principal component as the reference for the identification and determination of each known impurity in the routine analysis. However, if the correction factor is less than 0. 2 or more than 5, this method should be replaced by the reference substance method to avoid any error.

c. Main component self – control method without the corrected factor　Method: During the determination of any impurity, the drug reference substance solution or the diluted sample solution is used as the impurity reference solution. Measure the peak area of the impurity in the sample solution and the peak area of the principal component in the reference solution. The concentration of impurity in the sample solution is calculated as same as in the reference substance method.

This method is appropriate when the corrected factor is between 0. 9 ~ 1. 1 and out of this range, the corrected factor cannot be ignored during the calculation of the impurity content. Besides, for the unknown structure or unknown source impurities, this method seems the only way for the impurity control. However, if the unknown impurity content in drug is more than 0. 2% , the structure of this impurity should be identified. It is also encouraged to obtain the reference standard of the impurity and measure the corrected factor.

d. Peak area normalization method　Method：During the determination of the impurity content，inject the sample solution into the chromatography system and record the chromatogram. Measure the area of each peak and the total peak area except the solvent peak. Then calculate the percent of each impurity in the chromatogram for the limit control.

This method is simple and fast，however，there may be a large quantitative error when the impurity structure differs greatly from the principal component. Therefore，the Chinese Pharmacopoeia stated that this method cannot be used for the trace impurities test unless otherwise specified. This method only can be used for the situation that a high impurity content can be tolerated in drug.

6. 3 System suitability test

When using chromatographic method，the operator must confirm the chromategraphy system and operating procedures to ensure the accuracy of the data before analyzing the sample，which is depending on the system suitability test. To carry out the system suitability test，specific control substance is used to test and adjust the instrument to make sure the system meets the requirements；Or specify the minimum theoretical plates number，resolution，repeatability and trailing factors of the column during the analysis.

实验八　梯度洗脱法测定蒿甲醚中的有关物质

【实验目的】

1. 学习高效液相色谱中梯度洗脱法的原理。
2. 学习高效液相色谱法的条件优化方法。
3. 学习药物中有关物质测定的意义。

【实验原理】

1. 蒿甲醚的合成方法　蒿甲醚是青蒿素的重要衍生物之一，临床上是一种高效的抗疟药。蒿甲醚的常用制备方法（图 8 - 1）是将青蒿素通过硼氢化钠还原得到双氢青蒿素，进而在酸催化下将其与甲醇反应，得到蒿甲醚，最后通过重结晶提纯。青蒿素与双氢青蒿素分别是蒿甲醚的反应起始物和反应中间体，疏水性要弱于蒿甲醚，同时蒿甲醚合成过程中亦可能产生疏水性较强的反应副产物，需要采用相应的色谱方法对上述有关物质进行测定与控制，以确保蒿甲醚的药品质量。

2. 梯度洗脱　高效液相色谱的洗脱方式可以分为等度洗脱和梯度洗脱。等度洗脱指的是流动相的组成在整个色谱分析过程中不发生变化。而梯度洗脱指的是在色谱运行起始时间使用洗脱能力较弱的流动相，随着色谱运行时间的增加，流动相洗脱能力不断增强。

梯度洗脱可以避免等度洗脱的以下缺点：保留值 k 较小的组分洗脱时间过短，

扫码"学一学"

扫码"看一看"

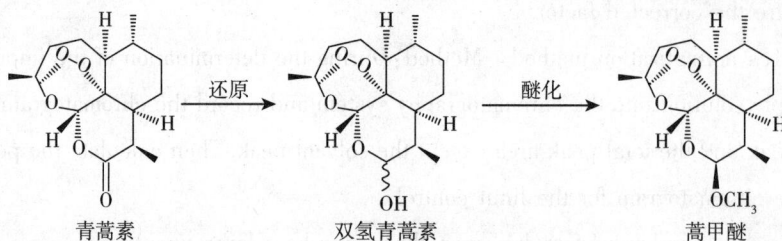

图 8-1 蒿甲醚的合成方法

甚至接近死时间，难以实现定量分析，造成色谱峰密集，分离度下降；而 k 值大的组分洗脱时间过长，造成峰展宽，柱效下降，甚至难以分辨；一些强保留的组分可能滞留在色谱柱上，不易被洗脱下来。在药物的有关物质控制中，可能不同有关物质的保留值差别较大，导致采用单一的等度洗脱方式无法进行同时洗脱。因此随着高效液相色谱仪器的普及，梯度洗脱方法已经逐渐成为药物的有关物质控制中主要的洗脱方式。

【仪器与试剂】

1. 仪器 高效液相色谱仪，紫外检测器，分析天平，液相微量进样针（100μl），量瓶（50ml、100ml），移液管（5ml）。

2. 试剂 青蒿素对照品（中国食品药品检定研究院），双氢青蒿素对照品（中国食品药品检定研究院），蒿甲醚原料药（自制），甲醇、乙腈为色谱级试剂，水为去离子水。

【实验内容】

1. 系统适用性溶液的配制 精密称取青蒿素和双氢青蒿素对照品适量，加入甲醇超声溶解，配制成含有青蒿素和双氢青蒿素浓度均为 1.0mg/ml 的系统适用性溶液。

2. 供试品溶液和对照溶液的配制 取蒿甲醚约 50mg，精密称定，置 50ml 量瓶中，加入乙腈溶解并稀释至刻度，摇匀，作为蒿甲醚供试品溶液（1.0mg/ml）。

定量移取蒿甲醚供试品溶液 5ml，置 100ml 量瓶中，用乙腈稀释配制成 50μg/ml 的对照溶液。

3. 色谱条件的设置 Baseline C_{18}（250mm×4.6mm×5μm）或同类型色谱柱；柱温：室温；流速：0.6ml/min；进样量：20μl；检测波长：216nm。

水为流动相 A，乙腈为流动相 B，按照下表进行梯度洗脱：

时间（min）	流动相 A（%）	流动相 B（%）
0	40	60
17	40	60
30	0	100
31	40	60
40	40	60

4. 系统适用性实验 精密量取系统适用性溶液 20μl，注入液相色谱仪，记录色谱图，调节起始流动相比例，使得青蒿素色谱峰保留时间为 10 分钟左右，α-双氢青蒿素和

β-双氢青蒿素相对于青蒿素的保留时间分别为 0.6 和 0.8，各峰之间分离度应大于 2.0。

5. 有关物质测定 精密量取蒿甲醚供试品溶液和对照溶液各 20μl，分别注入液相色谱仪，记录色谱图。供试品溶液谱图中如有杂质峰，其峰面积在对照溶液主峰面积 0.5~1.0 倍之间的杂质峰不得多于 1 个，其他单个杂质峰面积不得大于对照溶液主峰面积的 0.5 倍，各杂质峰面积的和不得大于对照溶液主峰面积的 2 倍（0.2%）。

【数据记录与处理】

1. 称样记录

表 8-1 称样记录

青蒿素的称样量	双氢青蒿素的称样量	供试品的称样量

2. 系统适用性实验结果

表 8-2 适用性实验结果

	保留时间	理论塔板数	对称因子	分离度
a-双氢青蒿素				
b-双氢青蒿素				
青蒿素				

3. 有关物质测定结果

表 8-3 有关物质测定结果

	主峰	杂质 1	杂质 2	杂质 3	杂质 4	总和
对照溶液		NA	NA	NA	NA	
供试品溶液	NA					
含量（%）	NA					

【讨论与指导】

1. 高效液相色谱分离条件的优化 高效液相色谱可供选择的分离条件主要是色谱柱固定相的种类和流动相的组成。

最常用的高效液相色谱色谱柱是反相色谱柱，即以 C_{18}（ODS 柱）、C_8、苯基等非极性官能团作为固定相的色谱柱，采用反相色谱柱，亲水性强（极性大）的物质出峰快，疏水性强（极性小）的物质出峰较慢。反相色谱系统的流动相常用甲醇-水系统和乙腈-水系统，当流动相中水相比例增加时，待测物在固定相上保留增强，分离度增加，但是水相比例过高可能导致峰型展宽反而降低分离度，一般反相流动相中有机溶剂比例不低于 5%。对于弱酸或弱碱性化合物，流动相中的添加剂（酸、碱、缓冲盐）浓度、种类和流动相 pH 也是重要的优化分离条件。在等度洗脱方式无法获得满意分离效果时，采用梯度洗脱方式可能获得较好的分离效果。

而正相色谱系统的固定相主要包括硅胶、二醇基等，流动相常用烷烃加适量极性调节剂而构成，如正己烷－异丙醇系统等。

2. 高效液相色谱检测条件的选择　高效液相色谱最常用的检测器为紫外－可见分光检测器（简称紫外检测器），包括二极管阵列检测器，其他常见的检测器有荧光检测器、蒸发光散射检测器、示差折光检测器、电化学检测器和质谱检测器等。

紫外－可见分光检测器、荧光检测器、电化学检测器为选择性检测器，其响应值不仅与被测物质的量有关，还与其结构有关；蒸发光散射检测器和示差折光检测器为通用检测器，对所有物质均有响应，结构相似的物质在蒸发光散射检测器的响应值几乎仅与被测物质的量有关。常用的检测器与被测物质的量在一定范围内呈线性关系，但蒸发光散射检测器的响应值与被测物质的量通常呈指数关系，一般需经对数转换。

流动相的选择常与检测器的类型密切相关，如反相色谱系统的流动相常用甲醇－水系统和乙腈－水系统，用紫外末端波长（205nm 以下）检测时，由于甲醇有较强的紫外吸收，宜选用乙腈－水系统；采用蒸发光散射检测器时，流动相中不能添加非挥发性的缓冲盐；采用示差折光检测器时，流动相不能使用梯度洗脱。

3. 梯度洗脱注意事项　虽然梯度洗脱已经成为药物有关物质测定中的最为常用的方式，但为获得理想的梯度洗脱分离效果和良好的重现性，在实验中必须考虑以下问题。

（1）滞留体积的影响　由于实现梯度洗脱的仪器设备结构或电子控制系统等多种原因，使得仪器系统中存在一定的滞留体积，不同仪器的结构和电路控制的差异，使其表现出的梯度洗脱系统的滞留时间不同，由滞留时间造成的保留时间和分离度的差别也不同。

（2）分离重现性　在梯度洗脱时，柱平衡是指用起始流动相冲洗色谱柱达到两相平衡。一个周期梯度洗脱结束时，流动相的组成与梯度洗脱起始时已大不相同，为了进行下一次梯度洗脱，必须用起始流动相对色谱柱彻底平衡后，再重新开始梯度洗脱。如果色谱柱未达到平衡，色谱图中洗脱较早的峰的保留值和分离度可能有变动。洗脱结束后，至少需要 $15 \sim 20$ 倍柱死体积的起始流动相充分洗脱后才可达到柱平衡，达到平衡所需流动相体积因溶剂和样品而异，需通过实验确定。

（3）基线问题　在样品进行梯度分离之前，必须进行一次空白梯度，即不注入样品，仅按梯度洗脱程序运行。空白梯度实验是在与样品梯度洗脱程序完全相同的条件下进行的，此时主要考察基线漂移和杂质峰。在梯度洗脱中，基线漂移是常见的现象，其中一种是由于 A 和 B 溶剂的紫外吸收不同造成的。在梯度洗脱中，有机溶剂 B 的浓度逐渐增加，通常有机溶剂如甲醇的紫外吸收大于水的吸收，因而若在梯度洗脱中使用紫外检测器，基线向上漂移是很普遍的现象，检测波长较低时这种现象更为严重。

Experiment 8　Determination of Related Substances in Artemether by the Gradient Elution

1. Experimental purposes

1. 1 To learn the principle of the gradient elution method in HPLC.

1. 2 To learn the opimization of the HPLC conditions.

1. 3 To learn the significance of related substances test in artemether.

2. Experimental principles

2.1 Synthesis method of artemether

Artemether is one of the important derivatives of artemisinin, which clinically used to treat malaria with high efficiency. The synthesis method of artemether usually including two steps: artemisinin is reduced by sodium borohydride to obtain dihydroartemisinin firstly, then the product reacted with methanol under acid catalysis to produce artemether. The final artemether can be purified by recrystallization. Artemisinin and dihydroartemisinin are the initial reactant and intermediate of respectively artemether, which have the less hydrophobicity than artemether. There are also some by-products with the high hydrophobicity during the synthesis of artemether. Therefore, it is necessary to control these related substances to ensure the quality of artemether.

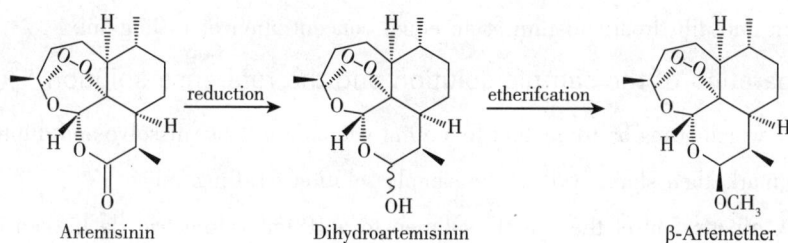

Fig. 8 – 1 Thesynthesis method of artemether.

2.2 Gradient elution

There are isometric and gradient elution methods for high performance liquid chromatography. For the isocratic elution, the compositions of the mobile phase keep constant throughout the chromatographic procedure. The gradient elution means that a weak elution strength of the mobile phase is used at the beginning and the elution strength increases during the analysis. Compare to the isocratic elution, the gradient elution avoids the following disadvantages: ① The elution time of the component with a small retention factor k is too short to close to the dead time of the column. It is difficult to achieve quantitative analysis, resulting in dense peaks and decreased resolution. ② On the other hand, the elution time of component with a large k value is too long to make peak broaden and the column efficiency decline to be indistinguishable. ③ Some strongly retained components may remain on the column and are not easily eluted.

For the control of related substances in drugs, the retention factors of various related substances may quite different each other, which result in the difficulty to be eluted by the isocratic elution. Therefore, with the popularization of HPLC instruments, the gradient elution has gradually become the main elution method in the control of related substances.

3. Apparatus and Reagents

3.1 Apparatus

High performance liquid chromatography; Ultraviolet detector; Analytical balance; Manual injection syringe for HPLC (100μl); Volumetric flask (50ml, 100ml); Transfer pipettes (5ml).

3. 2 Reagents

Artemisinin reference substance (National Institute for the Control of Pharmaceutical and Biological Products) ; Dihydroartemisinin reference substance (National Institute for the Control of Pharmaceutical and Biological Products) ; Artemether (Preparation in lab) ; Methanol and acetonitrile is the HPLC grade reagent and the other reagents are analytical reagent (AR) ; Water is deionized.

4. Experimental contents

4. 1 Preparation of the system suitability test solution

Accurately weigh an appropriate amount of artemisinin and dihydroartemisinin reference substance , dissolve them in methanol ultrasonically to prepare the system suitability test solution containing artemisinin and dihydroartemisinin at an equal concentration of 1. 0mg/ml.

4. 2 Preparation of the sample solution and the reference solution

Accurately weigh 50mg of artemether to a 50ml volumetric flask , dissolve and dilute it with acetonitrile to the mark , then shake well as the sample solution (1. 0mg/ml).

Accurately pipette 5ml of the sample solution to a 100ml volumetric flask , then dilute it with acetonitrile to the mark and shake well as the reference solution (50μg/ml).

4. 3 Setting of high performance liquid chromatography conditions

Baseline C_{18} (250mm × 4. 6mm × 5μm) or similar chromatographic column is used as the stationary phase. The column temperature is room temperature and the flow rate is 0. 6ml/min. The detection wavelength is 216nm and the inject volume is 20μl.

Mobile phase A , ultrapure water ; mobile phase B , acetonitrile. Gradient elution is performed according to the following table :

Time , min	Mobile phase A , %	Mobile phase B , %
0	40	60
17	40	60
30	0	100
31	40	60
40	40	60

4. 4 System suitability test

Inject 20μl of the system suitability test solution into the high perfor – mance liquid chromatography system and record the chromatogram. Adjust the ratio of the beginning mobile phase to make the retention time of artemisinin at approximately 10min , and the retention times of α – dihydroartemisinin and β – dihydroartemisinin relative to artemisinin are 0. 6 and 0. 8 , respectively. The resolution factor of each peak should be greater than 2. 0.

4. 5 Determination of related substances in artemether

Inject 20μl of the sample solution and the reference solution respectively into the high perfor mance liquid chromatography system and record the chromatograms. If there are impurities in the chromatogram of the sample solution, the number of impurity peaks with the peak area between 0. 5 and 1. 0 times of the main peak area in the reference solution is no more than one, the peak area of other single impurities is no more than 0. 5 times of the main peak area in the reference solution, and the sum of the areas of all impurity peaks is no more than twice of the main peak in the reference so-lution (0. 2%).

5. Data record and processing

5. 1 Record for the weight

Table 8 – 1　Record for the weight

Weight of artemisinin	Weight of dihydroartemisinin	Weight of the sample

5. 2 System suitability test

Table 8 – 2　System suitability test

	Retention time, (min)	Theoretical plates number	Symmetry factor	Resolution
α – dihydroartemisinin				
β – dihydroartemisinin				
Artemisinin				

5. 3 The results for the determination of related substances

Table 8 – 3　The results for the determination of related substances

	Main peak	Impurity peak 1	Impurity peak 2	Impurity peak 3	Impurity peak 4	Sum
The reference solution		NA	NA	NA	NA	
The sample solution	NA					
Percentage (%)	NA					

6. Discussion and guidance

6. 1 Optimization of HPLC separation conditions

The separation conditions of HPLC include the types of stationary phase and the composition of mobile phase.

The most commonly used HPLC column is the reversed phase chromatographic column, inclu-ding C_{18} (ODS), C_8, phenyl group and other nonpolar functional groups as the stationary phase. In the reversed phase chromatography, hydrophilic compound with large polarity elute earlier, while hydro phobic substances with small polarity elute later. Methanol/acetonitrile – water system is widely used as the mobile phase in the reversed phase chromatography. When the ratio of water increases, the retention of analyte on the stationary phase becomes strong and the resolution increases. However, too higher amount of water may lead to the peak broaden and lose resolution. Generally, there should be at least 5% of the organic solvent in the mobile phase of reversed phase chromatography. For the weakly acidic or basic compounds, the concentration and type of additives (acid, base, buffer salt) and the pH of mobile phase are also important optimized separation conditions. Using gradient elution method may get better result if isocratic elution method cannot get satisfactory separation.

The stationary phase of the normal phase chromatography system mainly includes silica gel and diol group, etc. The mobile phase usually composes of alkane and an appropriate amount of polarity regulator, such as the n – hexane – isopropanol system.

6. 2 Selection of detector for HPLC

The most commonly used detector for HPLC is ultraviolet – visible detector (UV – Vis), also called as UV detector, including diode array detectors (DAD). Besides that, fluorescence detector (FLD), evaporative light scattering detector (ELSD), refractive index detector (RID), electrochemical detect (ECD) and mass spectrometer detector (MSD) are also used in HPLC system.

The UV – Vis, FLD and ECD are selective detectors, the response value is not only related to the concentration of the analyte, but also related to its structure; ELSD and RID are common detectors that respond to all the compounds. For the ELSD, the response value of a similarly structured substance is almost only related to the concentration of the analyte. There is a linear relationship with the concentration of the analyte and the response value for most detectors. However, in the ELSD, the response value is generally exponential with the amount of the analyte and logarithmic conversion is usually necessary.

The mobile phase is closely related to the type of detector, such as methanol – water and acetonitrile – water are two commonly systems used in reversed phase chromatography. When using ultraviolet end wavelength (below 205nm); acetonitrile – water system is a better selection since methanol has strong ultraviolet absorption below 205nm. When using ELSD, non – volatile buffer salts cannot be added in the mobile phase. Gradient elution cannot be used when RID is selected as the detector.

6. 3 Notes for use of the gradient elution

Gradient elution has become the most commonly used method for the determination of related substances in drugs. In order to obtain the ideal separation effect and good reproducibility, the following issues should be considered.

a. Influence of hold – up volume   There is a certain retarded volume in the instrument due to the instrument structure or electronic control system for the gradient elution. Since the structure and circuit control of instruments are different, the hold – up time, the retention time and the resolution are also different.

b. Separation reproducibility   In the gradient elution, column equilibrium is achieved by flushing the column with the initial mobile phase to make the equilibrium between the two phases. At the end of a periodic gradient elution, the composition of the mobile phase is quite different from the beginning. For the next gradient elution, the initial flow must be thoroughly equilibrated relative to the column before the gradient elution is restarted. If the column is not completely equilibrious, the retention time and the resolution of the earlier eluted peaks may vary. Column equilibrium can only be achieved through fully eluted by at least $15 \sim 20$ times of dead volume of the initial mobile phase at the end of the elution. The volume of the mobile phase needed to achieve equilibrium may vary with the solvent and analyte, which should be determined through experiments.

c. Baseline issues　Before the analysis by the gradient elution, a blank gradient should be performed firstly, which means running the system according to the gradient elution program without injecting the analyte. The blank gradient experiment is performed under exactly the same conditions as the gradient elution procedure for sample analysis, where the baseline drift and impurity peaks are primarily investigated. Baseline drift is a common phenomenon in gradient elution, one of which is due to the different UV absorption of solvent A and solvent B. In the gradient elution, the concentration of the organic solvent B gradually increases, the ultraviolet absorption of an organic solvent such as methanol is usually greater than water. Therefore, baseline drift is a common phenomenon in UV detector system, especially under lower wavelength.

实验九　离子对色谱法测定利塞膦酸钠片含量的验证

【实验目的】

1. 学习含量测定方法学验证的项目。
2. 学习固体制剂含量测定的步骤。
3. 学习反相离子对色谱法的原理。

【实验原理】

1. 利塞膦酸钠片　利塞膦酸钠片中主要成分为利塞膦酸钠，其结构如图 9 - 1 所示。利塞膦酸钠片主要用于治疗和预防绝经后妇女的骨质疏松症。在绝经后骨质疏松的妇女中，利塞膦酸钠片可降低脊椎骨折的发生率，并可作为非脊椎骨质疏松相关骨折的复合用药。对于骨质疏松症的男性患者可有效增加其骨量。同时利塞膦酸钠片可以治疗和预防男性、女性糖皮质激素诱导的骨质疏松。此外还可以治疗变形性骨炎。服用这种药物的时候要注意不易和阿司匹林及非甾体类抗炎药一同服用，肾功能损害者应该慎用。

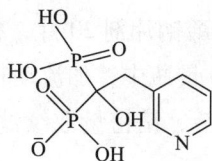

图 9 - 1　利塞膦酸钠的结构

2. 反相离子对色谱法的原理 反相离子对色谱法是把离子对试剂加到极性流动相中，被分析的样品离子在流动相中与离子对试剂（反离子）生成不带电荷的中性离子对，从而增加了样品离子在非极性固定相中的溶解度，使分配系数增加，改善分离效果。

对于碱性化合物（B），一般用各种烷基磺酸盐（$R-SO_3Na$）作离子对试剂，流动相和固定相之间的反应如图 9-2 所示。

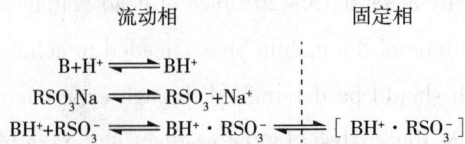

流动相   固定相

$$B+H^+ \rightleftharpoons BH^+$$
$$RSO_3Na \rightleftharpoons RSO_3^- + Na^+$$
$$BH^+ + RSO_3^- \rightleftharpoons BH^+ \cdot RSO_3^- \rightleftharpoons [BH^+ \cdot RSO_3^-]$$

图 9-2 碱性化合物形成离子对示意图

对于酸性化合物（RCOOH），一般用各种季铵盐，如四丁基铵类（TBA^+X^-），作离子对试剂，流动相和固定相之间的反应如图 9-3 所示。

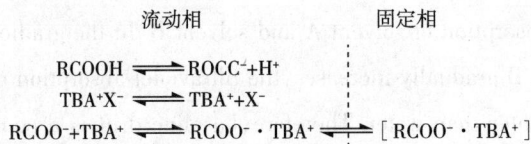

流动相   固定相

$$RCOOH \rightleftharpoons ROCC^+ + H^+$$
$$TBA^+X^- \rightleftharpoons TBA^+ + X^-$$
$$RCOO^- + TBA^+ \rightleftharpoons RCOO^- \cdot TBA^+ \rightleftharpoons [RCOO^- \cdot TBA^+]$$

图 9-3 酸性化合物形成离子对示意图

当中性离子对在固定相和流动相之间分配平衡之后，分配系数与离子对试剂碳链长度及分析物极性等因素有关。离子对试剂碳链长度越长，分配系数越大，保留时间越长。在反相离子对色谱中，流动相的 pH、离子对试剂的种类和浓度、有机溶剂的种类和浓度、缓冲盐、柱温等因素都会对分离产生很大影响。

【仪器与试剂】

1. 仪器 高效液相色谱仪，紫外检测器，分析天平，液相微量进样针（100μl），量瓶（25ml、50ml、100ml），移液管（5ml、10ml）。

2. 试剂 利塞膦酸钠片（市售品，5mg/片），利塞膦酸钠对照品（中国食品药品检定研究院），利塞膦酸钠片空白辅料（根据片剂处方配制），甲醇为色谱级试剂，其余试剂为分析纯，水为去离子水。

【实验内容】

1. 对照品溶液的配制 取利塞膦酸钠对照品约 20mg，精密称定，置 100ml 量瓶中，加流动相适量，振摇使溶解并稀释至刻度，摇匀，作为对照品储备液。精密量取对照品储备液 5ml，置 50ml 量瓶中，加流动相稀释至刻度，摇匀，作为对照品溶液。

2. 供试品溶液的配制 取利塞膦酸钠片剂 20 片，精密称定，研细，精密称取细粉适量（相当于利塞膦酸钠约 5mg），置 50ml 量瓶中，加流动相约 40ml，振摇使利塞膦酸钠溶解并稀释至刻度，摇匀，滤过，弃去初滤液，精密量取续滤液 5ml，置 25ml 量瓶中，加流动相稀释至刻度，摇匀，作为供试品溶液。

3. 色谱条件的设置 色谱柱：ODS 柱（250mm×4.6mm×5μm）或同类型色谱柱；流动相：甲醇-水（含 5mmol/L 磷酸二氢铵，2mmol/L 四丁基溴化铵，1.5mmol/L 乙二胺四乙酸二钠,用氢氧化钠溶液调节 pH 至 7.2)(25:75,*v/v*);柱温:室温;流速:1ml/min;进样量:20μl;检测波长:262nm;理论塔板数按利塞膦酸钠峰计算不低于 4000。

4. 专属性试验 取处方量辅料适量(相当于 20 片药品),按供试品溶液的配制操作,作为空白辅料溶液。精密量取空白辅料溶液 20μl 注入液相色谱仪,记录色谱图。另精密量取利塞膦酸钠对照品溶液 20μl 注入液相色谱仪,记录色谱图。观察辅料对利塞膦酸钠的测定是否产生干扰。

5. 标准曲线的制备 精密量取对照品储备液各 2、4、5、6、8ml,分别置 50ml 量瓶中,用流动相稀释至刻度,摇匀,作为系列对照品溶液。精密量取系列对照品溶液各 20μl 注入液相色谱仪,测定利塞膦酸钠峰面积。以系列对照品溶液的浓度(C)为横坐标,利塞膦酸钠的峰面积(A)为纵坐标进行线性回归,得标准曲线和回归方程。

6. 回收率试验 精密称取处方量辅料(相当于 20 片药品)九份,分别置于研钵中,精密称取利塞膦酸钠对照品 80、100 和 120mg 各三份,加入其中,混匀,研细。

分别称取上述细粉适量(相当于利塞膦酸钠约 5mg),按供试品溶液的配制操作,作为回收率试验样品。精密量取回收率试验样品各 20μl,分别注入液相色谱仪中,记录利塞膦酸钠的峰面积(A_1)。另精密量取对照品溶液 20μl,注入液相色谱仪中,记录利塞膦酸钠的峰面积(A_2)。按外标法以峰面积计算回收率试验样品的测得量,根据加入量和测定量的比值计算回收率。

7. 稳定性试验 供试品溶液室温放置 0、2、4、6、8、12、24 小时,各时间点精密量取 20μl,注入液相色谱仪中,测定峰面积,计算峰面积 *RSD* 值,*RSD* 值小于 2% 视为稳定性良好。

8. 重复性试验 取同一批片剂,制备六份供试品溶液,分别测定标示百分含量,计算标示百分含量之间的 *RSD* 值,*RSD* 值小于 2% 视为重复性良好。

9. 含量测定 精密量取供试品溶液 20μl,注入液相色谱仪,记录色谱图;另取对照品溶液 20μl,同法测定。按外标法以峰面积计算,即得利塞膦酸钠片的标示量百分含量。

【数据记录与处理】

1. 溶液的配制记录

表 9-1 对照品溶液的配制记录

对照品称样量(mg)	对照品储备液浓度(μg/ml)	对照品溶液浓度(μg/ml)

表 9-2 供试品溶液的配制记录

批号	20 片药品重量(g)	平均片重(mg)	取样量(mg)

2. 专属性试验图谱

（1）空白辅料色谱图

（2）对照品溶液色谱图

3. 回归方程的计算

表9-3　回归方程的原始数据记录和计算结果

系列对照品溶液峰面积					回归方程	相关系数
1	2	3	4	5		

4. 回收率试验结果

表9-4　回收率试验中对照品溶液的原始数据

	峰面积（A_1）		
	1	2	3
对照品溶液			

表9-5　回收率试验原始数据及计算结果

序号	加入量（mg）	峰面积（A_2）	测得量（mg）	回收率（%）	平均值（%）	RSD（%）
80%-1						
80%-2						
80%-3						
100%-1						
100%-2						
100%-3						
120%-1						
120%-2						
120%-3						

5. 稳定性试验结果

表9-6　稳定性试验原始数据及计算结果

	峰面积							RSD（%）
	0h	2h	4h	6h	8h	12h	24h	
供试品溶液								

6. 重复性试验结果

表 9 – 7 稳定性试验结果

	序号	峰面积	标示百分含量	RSD
供试品溶液	1			
	2			
	3			
	4			
	5			
	6			

7. 含量测定结果

表 9 – 8 含量测定结果

批号	峰面积	标示量的百分含量	平均值

【讨论与指导】

1. 含量测定方法学验证项目 含量测定方法验证的目的是证明采用的药物分析方法适合于相应的预期用途。每一种分析方法建立时需要根据分析目的进行验证，才能进行应用。药物中含量测定方法学验证的项目有：专属性、准确度、精密度、线性和线性范围、耐用性和稳定性等。专属性亦称选择性系指在其他成分（如杂质、降解物、辅料等）存在时，采用的分析方法能够准确分析待测物的能力，用于考察方法的抗干扰程度。如果专属性不佳，方法的准确度、精密度和线性都将受到影响。因此确保专属性是建立和验证一个分析方法的第一步。

2. 准确度与精密度 分析方法的准确度系指采用该方法测定的结果与真实值（可接受的约定真值或参考值）接近的程度，一般用回收率（%）表示。制剂的回收率测定可在处方量空白辅料中，加入已知量的被测物对照品进行测定。如不能得到制剂辅料（或中药），可向待测制剂（或中药）中加入已知量的被测物对照品进行测定。

精密度系指在规定的条件下，同一份均匀供试品，经多次取样测定所得结果之间的接近程度（分散度）。精密度一般用偏差、标准偏差或相对标准偏差表示。精密度可以从三个水平考虑：重复性、中间精密度和重现性。在相同条件下，由同一个分析人员测定所得结果的精密度称为重复性；在同一个实验室，不同时间由不同分析人员用不同设备测定结果之间的精密度，称为中间精密度；在不同实验室测定结果之间的精密度，称为重现性。

3. 线性和线性范围 线性系指在设计的测定范围内，检测结果与供试品中待测物浓度（或量）呈线性关系的程度。线性通常是制备一系列浓度的测试溶液（至少 5 种浓度）分析测定，以测得的信号响应值作为应变量，以待测物浓度作为自变量，以最小二乘法计算回归曲线。必要时，信号响应值可先经数学转换后，再进行线性回归计算。浓度与信号响应值（或响应值的数学转换形式）之间的线性相关程度，由相关系数表示。

4. 耐用性 系指在分析方法的参数发生微小的变化后，测定结果不受影响的能力，为所建立的方法用于日常检验提供可靠性依据。典型的变动因素有：被测溶液的稳定性、样品的提取次数、时间等。高效液相色谱法中典型的变动因素有：流动相的组成和 pH、不同品牌或不同批号的同类型色谱柱、柱温、流速等。气相色谱法变动因素有：不同品牌或批号的色谱柱、载气流速、柱温、进样口和检测器温度等。

Experiment 9 Validation for the assay of risedronate sodium tablets by ion – pair chromatography

1. Experimental Purposes

1.1 To learn the validation items for the assay.

1.2 To learn the procedures for assay of solid preparations.

1.3 To learn the principle for reversed phase ion – pair chromatography.

2. Experimental Principles

2.1 Risedronate sodium tablets

The main component of the risedronate sodium tablets is risedronate sodium and its structure is shown in Fig. 9 – 1. Risedronate sodium tablet is mainly applied for the treatment and prevention of osteoporosis in postmenopausal women. In postmeno – pausal women with osteoporosis, risedronate sodium tablets can reduce the incidence of spinal fractures and can be used as a kind of composite drug of non – vertebral osteoporosis – related fractures. It is also effective for the treatment to increase bone mass in male patients with osteoporosis. Meanwhile, risedronate sodium tablet is indicated for the treatment and prevention of glucocorticoid – induced osteoporosis in men and women. In addition, it can be applied for the treatment of Paget's disease of bone in men and women. It should not be taken with aspirin or non – steroidal anti – inflammatory drugs, and should be used with caution for people with kidney injury.

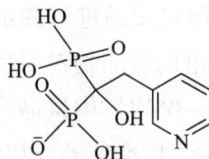

Fig. 9 – 1 The structure of risedronate sodium

2.2 Principle of reversed phase ion – pair chromatography

Reversed phase ion – pair chromatography involves the addition of an ion pair reagent to a polar mobile phase. Then a neutral ion pair without charge is formed by the analyte ion and the oppositely charged ion pair reagent in the mobile phase, thereby increasing the solubility of the ions in the non – polar stationary phase, which increases the distribution coefficient and improves the separation effect.

Foralkali compounds (B), the ion pair reagent is usually a kind of alkyl sulfonate ($R - SO_3$ Na). The reaction between the mobile phase and the stationary phase is shown in Fig. 9 – 2.

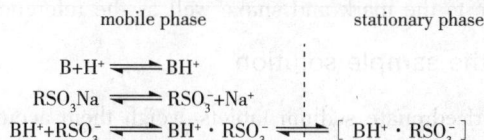

mobile phase　　　　　　stationary phase

$$B+H^+ \rightleftharpoons BH^+$$
$$RSO_3Na \rightleftharpoons RSO_3^- + Na^+$$
$$BH^+ + RSO_3^- \rightleftharpoons BH^+ \cdot RSO_3^- \rightleftharpoons [BH^+ \cdot RSO_3^-]$$

Fig. 9 – 2　Schematic diagram of alkali compounds forming ion pairs

For acidic compounds (RCOOH), the ion pair reagent is usually a kind of quaternary ammonium salt, such as tetrabutylammonium (TBA^+X^-). The reaction between the mobile phase and the stationary phase is shown in Fig. 9 – 3.

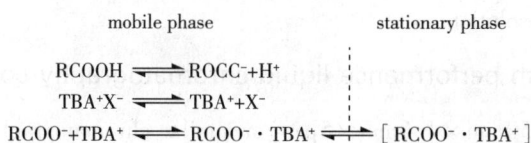

mobile phase　　　　　　stationary phase

$$RCOOH \rightleftharpoons ROCC^- + H^+$$
$$TBA^+X^- \rightleftharpoons TBA^+ + X^-$$
$$RCOO^- + TBA^+ \rightleftharpoons RCOO^- \cdot TBA^+ \rightleftharpoons [RCOO^- \cdot TBA^+]$$

Fig. 9 – 3　Schematic diagram of acidic compounds forming ion pairs

When the distribution of neutral ion pair is balanced between stationary phase and mobile phase, the distribution coefficient is related to the length of the carbon chain of the ion pair reagent and the polarity of the analytes. The longer the length of the carbon chain of the ion pair, the greater the distribution coefficient and the longer the retention time. In reversed – phase ion pair chromato – graphy, the factors, such as the pH of the mobile phase, the type and concentration of the ion pair reagent and organic solvent, the buffer salt, and the column temperature will all have a great influence on the separation.

3. Apparatus and Reagents

3. 1 Apparatus

High performance liquid chromatography; Ultraviolet detector; Analytical balance; Manual injection syringe for HPLC (100μl); Volumetric flask (25ml, 50ml, 100ml); Transfer pipettes (5ml, 10ml).

3. 2 Reagents

Risedronate sodium tablets (commercial products, 5mg/unit); Risedronate sodium reference substance (China National Institute for the Control of Pharmaceutical and Biological Products); The excipients of risedronate sodium tablets is prepared according to its prescription. Methanol is the HPLC grade reagent and the other reagents are analytical reagent (AR); Water is deionized.

4. Experimental contents

4. 1 Preparation of the reference solution

Accurately weigh 20mg of the risedronate sodium reference substance to a 100ml volumetric flask, dissolve and dilute it with the mobile phase to the mark, then shake well as the reference stock solution. Accurately pipette 5ml of the reference stock solution to a 50ml volumetric flask, then dilute it with the mobile phase to the mark and shake well as the reference solution.

4. 2 Preparation of the sample solution

Take 20 tablets of the risedronate sodium tablets, weigh them accurately and grind them finely. Then accurately weigh appropriate amount of powder (equivalent to about 5mg of risedronate sodium) to a 50ml volumetric flask. A 40ml of mobile phase is added to the volumetric flask and shake to dissolve the risedronate sodium. Then dilute it with the mobile phase to the mark and shake well. The solution is filtered and accurately pipette 5ml of the subsequent filtrate to a 25ml volumetric flask after discarding the initial filtrate. Then dilute it with the mobile phase to the mark and shake well as the sample solution.

4. 3 Setting of high performance liquid chromatography conditions

Lichrospher ODS (250mm × 4. 6mm × 5μm) or similar chromatographic column is used as the stationary phase. The mobile phase consisted of methanol : water (containing 5mmol/L ammonium dihydrogen phosphate, 2mmol/L tetrabutyl ammonium bromide and 1. 5mmol/L ethylenediamine tetraacetic acid disodium salt (EDTA − 2Na), adjust pH to 7. 2 with sodium hydroxide solution) (25 : 75, v/v) and the flow rat is 1. 0ml/min. The column temperature is room temperature. The detection wavelength is 262nm and the inject volume is 20μl. The number of theoretical plates is not less than 4000 according to the peak of risedronate sodium.

4. 4 Specificity

Weigh a quantity of excipients by prescription (equivalent to 20 tablets of the risedronate sodium tablets), then prepare the blank excipients solution according to the preparation procedure of the sample solution. Inject 20μl of the solution into the high performance liquid chromatography system and record the chromatograms. Inject another 20μl of the reference solution into the high performance liquid chromatography system and record the chromatograms. This experiment is used to investigate that whether interferences of excipients were found at the determination of risedronate sodium.

4. 5 Preparation of calibration curve

Accurately pipette 2, 4, 5, 6 and 8ml of the reference stock solution to the 50ml volumetric flask respectively, then dilute them with mobile phase to the mark and shake well as a series of reference solutions. Inject 20μl of each of the above solutions into the high performance liquid chromatography system and record the chromatograms. Then the peak area of the risedronate sodium was determined. The calibration curves and regression equation are performed by plotting the peak areas versus the corresponding concentrations.

4. 6 Recovery

Transfer a quantity of tablets excipients (equivalent to 20 tablets of risedronate sodium tablets, nine replicates) to the mortars respectively. Accurately weigh 80, 100 and 120mg of the risedronate sodium reference substance (three replicates respectively) to the mortars, mix and grind them well. Accurately weigh the appropriate amount of fine powder (equivalent to about 5mg of risedronate sodium), then prepare the recovery solutions according to the preparation procedure of the sample solution. Inject 20μl of the recovery solutions into the high performance liquid chromatography system respectively and record the chromatograms. Then inject 20μl of the reference solution for the assay of the sample by the external standard method according to the peak area of risedronate sodium and calculate the average recovery.

4. 7 Stability

Inject 20μl of the sample solution into the high performance liquid chromatography system at 0,2,4,6,8,12 and 24h respectively. Record the peak area and calculate the *RSD* value of peak areas. Stability is acceptable when *RSD* value is less than 2%.

4. 8 Repeatability

Transfer the same batch of tablets to prepare sample solutions (six replicates). Under the above chromatographic conditions,calculate the percentage of labelled amount and its RSD value. Repeatability is acceptable when the *RSD* value is less than 2%.

4. 9 Assay

Inject the sample solutions and record the chromatograms. Calculate the percentage of labelled amount by the external standard method according to the peak area of risedronate sodium.

5. Data recording and processing

5. 1 Record for the preparation of the solution

Table 9 − 1　Record for the preparation of the reference solution

The amount of reference substance (mg)	The concentration of the reference stock solution (μg/ml)	The concentration of the reference solution (μg/ml)

Table 9 − 2　Record for the preparation of the sample solutions

Batch number	Weight of 20 tablets(g)	Average weight of tablet(mg)	Sampling weight (mg)

5. 2 Chromatograms of the specificity

a. The chromatogram of the blank excipients

b. The chromatogram of the reference solution

5. 3 Calculation of regression equation

Table 9 – 3   The original data and calculation results of regression equation

Peak areas of a series of standard solutions					Regression equation	Correlation coefficient
1	2	3	4	5		

5. 4 The original data and calculation results of recovery

Table 9 – 4   The original data of the reference solutions in recovery test

	Peak area (A_1)		
	1	2	3
The reference solution			

Table 9 – 5   The original data and calculation results of recovery

Number	Added(mg)	Peak area(A_2)	Found(mg)	Recovery(%)	Ave(%)	RSD(%)
80% – 1						
80% – 2						
80% – 3						
100% – 1						
100% – 2						
100% – 3						
120% – 1						
120% – 2						
120% – 3						

5. 5 The original data and calculation results of stability

Table 9 – 6   The original data and calculation results of stability test

	Peak area							RSD (%)
	0h	2h	4h	6h	8h	12h	24h	
Sample solution								

5. 6 The original data and calculation results of repeatability

Table 9 – 7   The original data and calculation results of repeatability test

	Number	Peak area	The percentage of labelled amount	RSD
Sample solution	1			
	2			
	3			
	4			
	5			
	6			

5. 7 The original data and calculation results of assay

Table 9 – 8   The original data and calculation results of assay

Batch number	Peak area	The percentage of labelled amount	Ave

6. Discussion and guidance

6. 1 The validation items for the assay method

The validation for the assay method aims to confirming that the analytical method is suitable for its intended use. The analytical method needs to be verified before its use. The validation items for the assay includes specificity, accuracy, precision, linearity and range, stability and robustness.

The specificity also known as selectivity, refers to the ability to assess unequivocally the analyte in the presence of other components (impurities, degradants or matrix) which may be expected to be present. It is used to investigate the anti – interference level of the method. Lack of specificity of an analytical procedure may affect the accuracy, precision and linearity. Thus, the test of specificity is the first step in the establishment and validation of an assay method.

6. 2 Accuracy and precision

The accuracy of an analytical procedure is defined as the closeness of agreement between the value which is accepted either as a conventional true value or an accepted reference value and the value found. It is usually expressed by the recovery (%). The recovery of the preparation can be determined by adding a known amount of reference substance to the blank excipient. If the preparation excipients (or traditional Chinese medicine) cannot be obtained, a known amount of reference substance of analyte can be added to the preparation (or traditional Chinese medicine) for test.

The precision is defined as the closeness of agreement (degree of scatter) between a series of measurements obtained from multiple sampling of the same homogeneous sample under the prescribed conditions. Precision is usually expressed by deviation, standard deviation, or relative standard deviation. Precision may be considered at three levels: repeatability, intermediate precision, reproducibility. Repeatability expresses the precision measuring by the same analyst under the same operating conditions; intermediate precision expresses the precision measuring within – laboratories variations: different days, different analysts, different equipment, etc. ; reproducibility expresses the precision between laboratories.

6. 3 Linearity and range

The linearity is its ability (within a given range) to obtain test results which are keeping a linear relation to the concentration (amount) of analyte in the sample. Linearity is measured usually by a series of concentrations of the test solution (at least 5 levels), and calculate the regression equation by the linear least – squares regression with the measured signal response value as the dependent variable and the concentration as the independent variable. If necessary, the signal response value can be converted by mathematics before linear regression calculation. The extent of linear correlation between the concentration and the signal response value (or the mathematical conversion form of the response value) is expressed by the correlation coefficient.

6. 4 Robustness

The robustness is the capacity to remain unaffected by small, but deliberate variations in method parameters and provides an indication of its reliability during normal usage. The typical variation factors: the stability of the test solution, times of sample extraction, time, etc. The variation factors of HPLC include composition and pH value of mobile phase, chromatographic column of different brands or batches, column temperature, flow rate, etc. The variation factors of gas chromatography include chromatographic column of different brands or batches, flow rate of gas, column temperature, injection port and detector temperature.

扫码"学一学"

扫码"学一学"

实验十　手性高效液相色谱法拆分左氧氟沙星对映异构体

【实验目的】

1. 学习拆分对映异构体的目的。
2. 学习手性高效液相色谱法的分类。
3. 学习手性流动相添加剂法的拆分原理。

【实验原理】

1. 左氧氟沙星的性状　左氧氟沙星（Levofloxacin，图 10 − 1a）是一种氟喹诺酮类广谱抗细菌药，可用于治疗细菌性的鼻窦炎、肺炎、泌尿道感染、慢性前列腺炎以及肠胃炎等疾病。其纯品是类白色至淡黄色结晶性粉末，分子量为 361.37，在水中微溶，在乙醇中极微溶，在乙醚中不溶。左氧氟沙星属于手性药物，其分子结构中含有 1 个手性中心，可能存在 1 个对映异构体，即右氧氟沙星（图 10 − 1b）。对映异构体杂质无法采用常规的高效液相色谱分离控制，需要采用手性高效液相色谱法进行拆分。

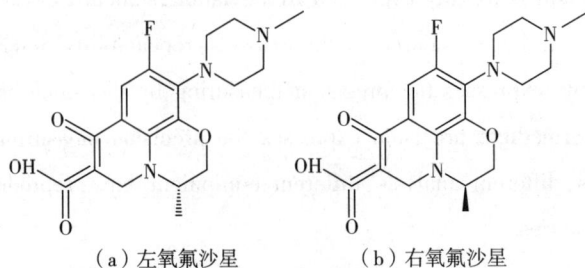

（a）左氧氟沙星　　　（b）右氧氟沙星

图 10 − 1　左氧氟沙星和右氧氟沙星的结构

2. 手性高效液相色谱法　分子组成相同，但空间结构上互为镜像关系（手性对称）的一对立体异构体称为对映异构体，简称对映体。虽然对映体的理化性质几乎完全相同，但是它们的药效学和药动学行为常有所不同，从而导致其药理和毒理作用有所差异。对于单一对映体药物，可能共存的另外一个对映异构体是其杂质之一，如左旋氧氟沙星中的右旋氧氟沙星杂质，因此需要对其进行限度控制。常规的高效液相色谱方法无法分离对映异构体，需要采用专门的手性高效液相色谱法进行对映异构体拆分。目前，手性高效液相色谱法可以分为手性衍生化试剂法、手性固定相法和手性流动相法。

对于喹诺酮类手性药物的拆分，以配基交换试剂作为手性流动相添加剂的手性高效液相色谱法较为常用。该法指在流动相中加入金属离子和配位体交换剂形成二元络合物，以适当的浓度分布于流动相中，遇到药物消旋体形成稳定性不同的三元络合物，在普通的反相键合色谱柱上达到手性分离。常用的手性配合试剂多为光学活性氨基酸及其衍生物，如 $L-$ 苯丙氨酸、$L-$ 脯氨酸等；配位金属有 Cu^{2+}、Zn^{2+}、Ni^{2+} 等。配基交换系统大多使用水性流动相和疏水固定相，如 C_{18}、C_8 柱。其交换机制可表示为：

$$[CL]_nM + [CS] \rightleftharpoons [CL]_{n-1}[M][CS] + [CL] \quad (n \geq 2)$$

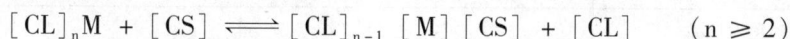

式中，CL 为手性配位体，M 为金属离子，$(CL)_nM$ 为所形成的络合物，CS 为 R- 和 $S-$ 或 $D-$ 和 $L-$异构体。

【仪器与试剂】

1. 仪器 高效液相色谱仪（配紫外检测器），分析天平，微量注射器（100μl），量瓶（10ml），移液管（2ml），液相手动进样针（100μl）。

2. 试剂 左氧氟沙星对照品（中国食品药品检定研究院）；右氧氟沙星对照品（中国食品药品检定研究院）；左氧氟沙星原料药（纯度>99%）；甲醇为色谱纯；硫酸铜、$D-$苯丙氨酸为分析纯试剂；水为超纯水。

【实验内容】

1. 对照品溶液的配制 取右氧氟沙星对照品约5mg，精密称定，加流动相溶解并定量逐级稀释制成每1ml约含10μg的溶液，作为右氧氟沙星对照溶液；精密量取该溶液适量，用流动相定量稀释制成每1ml中约含0.5μg的溶液，作为灵敏度溶液。

取左氧氟沙星对照品约10mg，精密称定，置10ml量瓶中，加流动相溶解并稀释至刻度，摇匀，作为左氧氟沙星对照溶液。

2. 供试品溶液的配制 取左氧氟沙星原料药约10mg，精密称定，置10ml量瓶中，加流动相溶解并稀释至刻度，摇匀，作为供试品溶液。

3. 色谱条件的设置 色谱柱：Zorbax SB-C_{18}（4.6mm×150mm×5μm）或同类型色谱柱；流动相：硫酸铜$D-$苯丙氨酸溶液（含1g硫酸铜与1.32g $D-$苯丙氨酸，加水1000ml溶解后，用氢氧化钠调节 pH 至3.5）-甲醇（82∶18，v/v）；检测波长：294nm；流速：1.0ml/min；柱温：45℃；进样量：10μl。

4. 流动相甲醇比例的优化 在20%~40%范围内选择设定不同的有机相比例，分别取10μl左氧氟沙星及右氧氟沙星对照品溶液注入液相色谱仪，记录依序出峰时间；取10μl样品溶液注入液相色谱仪，记录右氧氟沙星与相邻干扰色谱峰的分离度，选择分离度不小于1.2的流动相条件用于含量测定。

5. 系统适用性实验 取适量左氧氟沙星对照品和右氧氟沙星对照品，加流动相溶解并稀释制成每1ml中约含左氧氟沙星1mg、右氧氟沙星20μg的混合溶液，作为系统适用性溶液。取10μl注入液相色谱仪，记录色谱图，左氧氟沙星与右氧氟沙星的分离度应符合要求。取灵敏度溶液10μl注入液相色谱仪，主成分色谱峰峰高的信噪比应大于10。

6. 右氧氟沙星的检查　精密量取供试品溶液和右氧氟沙星对照溶液 $10\mu l$，分别注入液相色谱仪，记录色谱图。供试品溶液色谱图中右氧氟沙星峰面积不大于对照溶液主峰面积（1.0%）。

【数据记录与处理】

1. 溶液的配制记录

表 10－1　对照品溶液的配制记录

名称	称样量（W）	溶液浓度（C_S）
左氧氟沙星对照品		
右氧氟沙星对照品		
左氧氟沙星原料药		

2. 甲醇比例的优化结果

表 10－2　甲醇比例的优化结果

条件	保留时间/min		主峰理论塔板数	分离度
	左氧氟沙星	右氧氟沙星		
20%甲醇				
25%甲醇				
30%甲醇				
35%甲醇				
40%甲醇				

3. 系统适用性实验结果

表 10－3　系统适用性实验结果

	保留时间/min		分离度	信噪比
	左氧氟沙星	右氧氟沙星		
系统适用性溶液				NA
灵敏度溶液			NA	

4. 测定的原始数据

表 10－4　测定的原始数据

	序号	保留时间/min	峰面积	杂质含量
对照溶液	1			
	2			NA
	3			
供试品溶液	1			
	2			
	3			

【讨论与指导】

1. 手性流动相法的添加剂　在流动相中加入光学纯的手性添加剂，使其与待测物形成非对映异构复合物，根据其形成复合物的稳定常数不同而获得分离，具体有两种作用方式：①流动相中手性试剂与对映体形成非对映体配合物，在固定相中的保留时间和分配不同而得到拆分；②手性试剂吸附在柱上形成动态的手性固定相，对映异构体与之作用不同而得到拆分。常用的手性添加剂主要包括环糊精类、手性离子对试剂和配基交换型试剂三类。

本实验在流动相中加入硫酸铜 L – 苯丙氨酸溶液，属于配基交换型手性流动相法。分离时，手性配体交换剂先吸附在疏水性固定相表面（C_{18}）构成动态手性固定相，与对映体作用形成非对映异构体的配合物，经洗脱分离，顺序与一般反相高效液相色谱一致。流动相中加入乙腈或甲醇等有机改性剂，可缩短疏水性药物的保留时间，并提高分离度。

2. 影响手性流动相法拆分的因素　添加剂的种类和浓度、有机相的比例、流动相的 pH 等因素对手性拆分的效能、选择性和分离度都有很大的影响，应根据实验寻找最优值。

（1）添加剂的类型和浓度　以手性离子对试剂为例，不同的离子对试剂，其立体选择性不同，如 10 – 樟脑磺酸比 3 – 溴 – 10 – 樟脑磺酸的选择性大。此外，随着试剂浓度增加，对映体的拆分效果增强。

（2）有机溶剂　在反相色谱中，有机溶剂比例越大，对映体在色谱柱上保留时间越短，可以有效缩短分析时间；但是，有机溶剂含量过高，可能导致手性添加剂溶解度降低，如环糊精，从而显著影响对映体的分离度。

（3）pH　通常酸度增大，有利于碱性药物的分离。随 pH 的减小，容量因子先增大后减小，而分离度随酸度的增加而增大。

3. 三类手性液相色谱法的比较　手性液相色谱法包括柱前衍生化法、手性流动相法和手性固定相法三类。

（1）柱前衍生化法　是在进行色谱分离前，将手性药物对映体与高光学纯度的手性衍生化试剂进行反应，从而引入另一个手性中心，形成非对映异构体，再以常规 HPLC 进行分离。该方法采用价格便宜、柱效较高的非手性柱，通过在色谱分离前进行衍生化，纯化样本、引入发色基团，改善分离的同时可提高检测灵敏度；但是反应费时、操作繁琐亦是它的不足。

（2）手性流动相法　即在流动相中加入手性添加剂，使其与手性药物对映异构体形成非对映异构体复合物，根据复合物的稳定常数不同而获得分离。该方法操作简便，无需昂贵的手性柱、无需复杂的衍生化；但是可拆分的药物有限，且某些添加剂稳定性不佳，大量加入，亦会增加费用。

（3）手性固定相法　是基于手性药物对映异构体与固定相表面的手性选择剂形成暂时的非对映异构体配合物的能量差异或稳定性不同，达到手性分离的方法。适用于不含活泼反应基团的药物，同时无需高光学纯度试剂、样品处理简单，可实现制备分离；但是昂贵的价格在一定程度上制约了手性柱的广泛使用。

4. 手性杂质对药物质量的影响　手性药物的光学异构体不仅在药物活性上存在很大的差别，有的还会影响用药的安全性和有效性，如氧氟沙星外消旋体的药理作用仅为左旋体的一半；沙利度胺的 R – 体安全有效，而 S – 体及其代谢产物却有很强的致畸作用和胚胎毒性；止吐药扎考必利的两个光学异构体的药理作用完全相反，R – 体为 5 – HT_3 受体拮抗剂，而 S – 体为 5 – HT_3 受体激动剂。因此，建立良好的对映异构体分离及检查方法对保障相关药品质量具有重要意义。

Experiment 10   Resolution of the Enantiomer of Levofloxacin by Chiral High Performance Liquid Chromatography

1. Experimental purposes

1. 1 To learn the purpose of resolution of enantiomers.

1. 2 To learn the classification of chiral high performance liquid chromatography.

1. 3 To learn the principle of chiral mobile phase additives.

2. Experimental principles

2. 1 The characters of levofloxacin

Levofloxacin (Fig. 10 – 1a) is a broad – spectrum antibacterial fluoroquinolone that can be used to treat bacterial sinusitis, pneumonia, urinary tract infections, chronic prostatitis, and gastroenteritis. Its pure product is a white – like to pale yellow crystalline powder with a molecular weight of 361. 37, slightly soluble in water, very slightly soluble in ethanol, and insoluble in ether. Levofloxacin is a chiral drug with a chiral center in its molecular structure and has one enantiomer, R – ofloxacin (Fig. 10 – 1b). Chiral high – performance liquid chromatography (HPLC) is required since conventional HPLC is not capable of separating enantiomers.

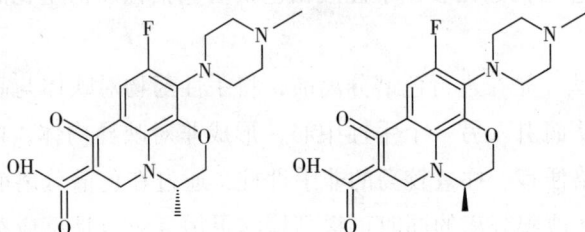

Fig. 10 – 1   Structures of (a) levofloxacin and (b) (R) – ofloxacin

2. 2 Chiral HPLC

Enantiomers are a pair of stereoisomers having the same molecular composition but are mirror images of each other. The different pharmacodynamic and pharmacokinetic behaviors make different pharmacological and toxicological effects, although the physicochemical properties of enantiomers are almost identical. For an enantiomeric drug, the existed enantiomer may be one of the impurities, such as the dextrofloxacin in levofloxacin. Therefore, the enantiomer should be controlled. Chiral HPLC is required since conventional HPLC cannot separate the enantiomers. At present, chiral HPLC includes chiral derivatization, chiral stationary phase and chiral mobile phase method.

Chiral HPLC with ligand exchange reagents as chiral mobile phase additives is commonly used for the resolution of quinolone chiral drugs. The added metal ion and the ligand exchanger could form the binary complex distributed in the mobile phase at an appropriate concentration. Enantiomers could form ternary complexes with them and achieve the chiral separation on a common reversed – phase bonded column according to the different stability of complexes. Commonly used chiral ligand exchange reagents are optically active amino acids and their derivatives, such as L – phenylalanine, L – valine, while coordination metals are Cu^{2+}, Zn^{2+}, Ni^{2+}, and the like. Most of the ligand exchange systems use aqueous mobile phases and hydrophobic stationary phases, such as C_{18} and C_8 columns. The exchange mechanism can be expressed as follows:

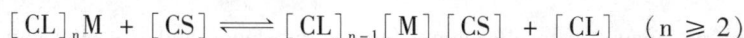

$$[CL]_nM + [CS] \rightleftharpoons [CL]_{n-1}[M][CS] + [CL] \quad (n \geqslant 2)$$

Where, CL is a chiral ligand, M is a metal ion, $[CL]_nM$ is a complex formed, and CS are a pair of stereoisomers.

3. Apparatus and Reagents

3.1 Apparatus

High performance liquid chromatograph system (with UV detector); Analytical balance; Microsyringe ($100\mu l$); Volumetric flask (10ml); Pipettes (2ml); Manual syringe for LC ($100\mu l$).

3.2 Reagents

Levofloxacin reference substance (National institute for the control of pharmaceutical and biological products); R – ofloxacin (National institute for the control of pharmaceutical and biological products); Levofloxacin (purity is more than 99%); Methanol is HPLC grade reagent; Copper sulfate and D – phenylalanine are analytical reagent (AR); Water is deionized.

4. Experimental contents

4.1 Preparation of the reference solution

Accurately weigh 5mg of the R – ofloxacin reference substance to a 10ml volumetric flask, then dissolve and stepwise dilute with the mobile phase to prepare the reference solution of R – ofloxacin ($10\mu g/ml$). Then accurately pipette amounts of the reference solution, and dilute it with the mobile phase to prepare the sensitivity solution of R – ofloxacin ($0.5\mu g/ml$).

Accurately weigh approximate 10mg of the levofloxacin reference substance to a 10ml volumetric flask, then dissolve and dilute it with the mobile phase, and shake well before use.

4.2 Preparation of the sample solution

Accurately weigh 10mg of levofloxacin bulk drug substance to a 10ml volumetric flask, then dissolve and dilute with mobile phase, and shake well before use.

4.3 HPLC conditions

Agilent Zorbax SB – C_{18} ($4.6mm \times 150mm$, $5\mu m$) or similar columns is used as the stationary phase. Copper sulfate D – phenylalanine solution (1g of copper sulfate and 1.32g of D – phenylalanine, dissolved in 1000ml of water, adjusted to pH 3.5 with sodium hydroxide) – methanol (82 : 18, v/v) are used as the mobile phase with the flow rate of 1.0ml/min and the column temperature of 45℃. The injection volume and detection wavelength are $10\mu l$ and 294nm, respectively.

4.4 Optimization of methanol ratio in the mobile phase

The methanol ratio in the mobile phase is optimized at the range from 20% to 40%. For each ratio, inject $10\mu l$ of the reference solution of levofloxacin and R – ofloxacin into the HPLC system, and record their retention times; inject $10\mu l$ of the sample solution into the HPLC system, and record the resolution between the chromatographic peak of R – ofloxacin and the adjacent peaks. The resolution should be no less than 1. 2 for the assay.

4. 5 System suitability

Take appropriate amount of levofloxacin reference substance and R – ofloxacin reference substance, dissolve and dilute them with the mobile phase to prepare the system suitability solution containing about 1mg/ml of levofloxacin and $20\mu g/ml$ of R – ofloxacin. Inject $10\mu l$ of the system suitability solution into the HPLC system, and record the peak response and retention time. The resolution between levofloxacin and R – ofloxacin complies with the related requirement. Inject $10\mu l$ of the sensitivity solution into the HPLC system, and the signal – to – noise ratio of the peak height of the main chromatographic peak should be greater than 10.

4. 6 Limit test for R – ofloxacin

Separately inject $10\mu l$ of the sample solution and the R – ofloxacin reference solution into the HPLC system, and record the chromatograms. The area of the R – ofloxacin peak in the chromatogram of the sample solution should not be larger than the area of the main peak in the chromatogram of the reference solution (1. 0%).

5. Data record and processing

5. 1 Record for the solution preparation

Table 10 – 1   Record for the solution preparation

Substance	Weight	Concentration
Levofloxacin reference substance		
R – ofloxacin reference substance		
Levofloxacin bulk drug substance		

5. 2 Optimization of methanol ratio

Table 10 – 2   Results of the optimization of methanol ratio

Condition	Retention time (min)		Theoretical plate number	Resolution
	Levofloxacin	R – ofloxacin		
20% methanol				
25% methanol				
30% methanol				
35% methanol				
40% methanol				

5. 3 System suitability

Table 10 – 3   Data of system suitability

	Retention time (min)		Resolution	S/N
	Levofloxacin	R – ofloxacin		
System suitability solution				NA
Sensitivity solution			NA	

5. 4 Original data of limit test

Table 10 – 4   The original data of limit test

	Number	Retention time (min)	Peak area	Content (%)
Reference solution	1			
	2			NA
	3			
Sample solution	1			
	2			
	3			

6. Discussion and guidance

6. 1 Additives of the chiral mobile phase method

The optically pure chiral additive is added to the mobile phase to form the diastereomeric complexes with the analytes, and the separation is obtained according to the different stability constants of the formed complexes. There are two mechanisms: ①the chiral reagents and enantiomers form the diastereomeric complexes in the mobile phase, and they are separated by their different retention times and distributions in the stationary phase; ②the chiral reagent is adsorbed on the column to form a dynamic chiral stationary phase, and the enantiomers are separated by their different effects with it. The commonly used chiral additives mainly include cyclodextrins, chiral ion – pairing reagents and ligand – exchangeable reagents.

In this experiment, the copper sulfate L – phenylalanine solution added in the mobile phase is a kind of the ligand – exchangeable reagents. The chiral ligand exchanger is first adsorbed on the surface of the hydrophobic stationary phase (C_{18}) to form a dynamic chiral stationary phase that interact with enantiomers to form the diastereomeric complexes. Then the complexes are separated by elution, and the elution sequence is consistent with that in the general reversed – phase HPLC.

6. 2 Factors affecting the separation in the chiral mobile phase method

Factors such as the types and concentrations of the additives, the ratio of the organic phase, and the pH of the mobile phase have a great influence on the efficiency, selectivity and resolution of the chiral separation. The optimum value should be found according to the optimization experiment.

a. Types and concentrations of additives   Taking chiral ion – pairing reagents as an example, different ion – pairing reagents have different stereoselectivity, such as 10 – camphorsulfonic acid having a greater selectivity than 3 – bromo – 10 – camphorsulfonic acid. In addition, the resolution of the enantiomer would be enhanced with the increased concentration of the reagents.

b. Organic solvent   In reversed – phase HPLC, the larger the proportion of organic solvent, the shorter the retention time of the enantiomers on the column, which can effectively shorten the analysis time. However, if the organic solvent content is too high, the solubility of some chiral additives (e. g. cyclodextrin) may decrease, which signifycantly affects the resolution of the enantiomers.

c. pH   Generally, the increase of acidity is beneficial to the separation of alkaline drugs. The capacity factor increases first and then decreases with the decreased pH, while the resolution increases.

6.3 Comparison of three types of chiral HPLC

Chiral HPLC includes the chiral derivatization method, the chiral stationary phase method and the chiral mobile phase method.

a. Chiral derivatization method   The chiral drug enantiomers are reacted with high optical purity chiral derivatization reagents to form the diastereomers before being separated by the conventional HPLC column. The conventional nonchiral column is cheap and high efficiency. The derivatization prior to chromatographic separation can purify the samples, introduce the chromophore group, improve the resolution and detection sensitivity. However, the operation procedure of derivatization is usually time – consuming and tedious.

b. Chiral mobile phase method   The chiral additive is added to the mobile phase to form the diastereomeric complexes with the chiral drug enantiomers, and the separation is obtained according to the different stability constants of the complexes. The method is simple and convenient, avoiding the expensive chiral columns and the complicated derivatization procedure. However, the drugs that can be analyzed by this method are limited, and the cost will increase if a large amount of additives were added to improve their poor stability.

c. Chiral stationary phase method   The chiral separation is achieved based on the differences in energy or stability of the temporary diastereomeric complexes formed by the chiral selector on the surface of the stationary phase and the chiral drug enantiomers. It is suitable for drugs without active reactive groups, and it does not require high optical purity reagents. Moreover, sample preparation is simple and preparative chromatography is available. However, the chiral column is expensive so this method is not universal.

6.4 Effect of chiral impurities on drug quality

The optical isomers of chiral drugs not only have great differences in drug activity, but also affect the safety and effectiveness of the drug. For example, the pharmacological action of ofloxacin racemate is only half of that of the left – handed one. The R – thalidomide is safe and effective, while the S – thalidomide and its metabolites have strong teratogenic effects and embryotoxicity. The pharmacological effects of the two optical isomers of zacopride, the antiemetic drug, are completely opposite. The R – zacopride is a $5 – HT_3$ receptor antagonist while the S – zacopride is a $5 – HT_3$ receptor agonist. Therefore, a good method for separation and detection of enantiomers is meaningful to ensure the quality of related drugs.

扫码"练一练"

第三章　色谱技术在药物鉴定中的应用

Chapter 3　Application of Chromatographic Techniques in the Drug Identification

扫码"学一学"

实验十一　薄层色谱法鉴定复方磺胺甲噁唑片中磺胺甲噁唑和甲氧苄啶

【实验目的】

1. 学习薄层色谱法的操作及原理。
2. 学习比移值 R_f 及分离度 R 的概念。
3. 学习薄层色谱法在药物分析中应用。

【实验原理】

1. 磺胺甲噁唑和甲氧苄啶的性质　磺胺甲噁唑（SMZ）是一种常用的磺胺类抗菌药物，具有较好的广谱抗菌消炎作用。其产品为白色结晶性粉末，密度 1.462，熔点 166 ~ 169℃，沸点 482℃，折射率 1.66。本品几乎不溶于水，略溶于乙醇，易溶于丙酮、稀氢氧化钠溶液和稀酸溶液。甲氧苄啶（TMP）为抗菌剂，抗菌范围和磺胺药相近，与磺胺类药物并用时具有明显增效作用，可增加十至数十倍的效果。其产品为白色结晶粉末，熔点 199 ~ 203℃。本品在水中几乎不溶，在三氯甲烷、乙醇或丙酮中微溶，在冰醋酸中易溶。

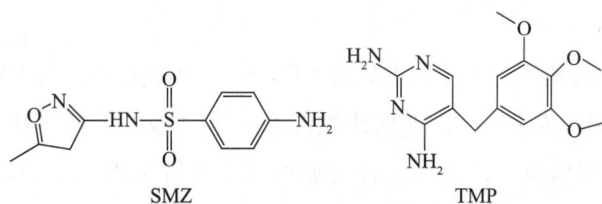

图 11 - 1　磺胺甲噁唑和甲氧苄啶结构式

2. 薄层色谱法原理　薄层色谱法是将固定相均匀涂布在表面光滑的平板上形成薄层，点样展开后，由于各组分与固定相和流动相的作用力大小不同，导致其在薄层板上的迁移速度和距离不一致而分离。比较其比移值（R_f）与同等条件下对照品的比移值（R_f），实现定性鉴别。

$$R_f = L / L_0$$

式中，L 为原点到组分斑点中心的距离；L_0 为原点到溶剂前沿的距离。

将复方磺胺甲噁唑供试品溶液及 SMZ 和 TMP 对照品溶液分别点样在硅胶 GF$_{254}$ 荧光板上，在三氯甲烷 – 甲醇 – 二甲基甲酰胺（20∶2∶1）溶液中展开，SMZ 和 TMP 受到硅胶对其不同的吸附力和展开剂对其不同的溶解度、色散力而达到分离，样品组分猝灭所在处的荧光而产生暗斑，并与同板上对照品暗斑进行比较，根据 R_f 进一步进行定性鉴别。

SMZ 和 TMP 的分离度按下式计算。

$$R = 2\,(L_2 - L_1)\,/\,(W_1 + W_2)$$

式中，L_1、L_2 分别为供试品中的两斑点的迁移距离；W_1、W_2 分别为供试品中的两斑点的纵向直径。

$R = 1.0$ 时，相邻两斑点基本分开。

【仪器与试剂】

1. 仪器　层析缸（20cm×20cm），玻璃板（20cm×5cm），紫外光照灯（254nm），点样毛细管（或微量注射器），小烧杯（或乳钵），玻璃棒，牛角匙等。

2. 试剂　复方磺胺甲噁唑片剂（市售，每片含 400mg 的 SMZ 和 80mg 的 TMP），SMZ、TMP 对照品（中国食品药品检定研究院），三氯甲烷 – 甲醇 – 二甲基甲酰胺（分析纯试剂，按体积比 20∶2∶1 配制），硅胶 GF$_{254}$，羧甲基纤维素钠（CMC – Na）水溶液（0.75g/100ml）。

【实验内容】

1. 对照品溶液的配制　分别精密称定 SMZ 对照品 0.2g、TMP 对照品 40mg，用 10ml 甲醇溶解，摇匀，备用。

2. 供试品溶液的配制　取磺胺甲噁唑片剂 10 片，研磨磨细，取适量磨细的粉末（约相当于 SMZ 0.2g），加 10ml 甲醇溶解，震荡后过滤，取续滤液作为供试品溶液。

3. 薄层色谱鉴别

（1）硅胶薄层板的制备　天平称取硅胶 GF$_{254}$ 6g 于小烧杯中。加 CMC – Na 水溶液 17ml（硅胶与黏合剂的比例约为 1∶3），玻璃棒搅拌 5 分钟（或在乳钵中研磨），将糊状的固定相转移至洗净晾干的玻璃板上，震动、转动玻璃板几分钟至板表面均匀平滑，将其水平放置通风处晾干，再在 110℃ 活化 1 小时，置于干燥器中备用。

（2）点样　在距板底边约 2.0cm 处用铅笔做一起始记号，用点样毛细管将 SMZ 对照品溶液、供试品溶液、TMP 对照品分别点样 5μl（约毛细管的 1cm）于薄层板，斑点直径不超过 3mm，挥干溶剂。

（3）展开　将 18ml（或适量）展开剂倒入双槽层析缸中的一侧内，将薄层板点有样品的一端朝下放入层析缸中的另一侧内，盖上磨砂玻璃盖密闭，饱和 10～15 分钟后，倾斜层析缸让展开剂流入放置薄层板的一侧（或直接将薄层板转移至展开剂的一侧），并浸入点样

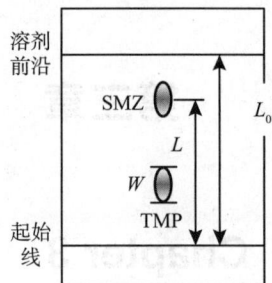

端0.3~0.5cm，待溶剂前沿展开约10cm时取出薄层板。

（4）显色和数据采集　取出薄层板后，迅速用铅笔标记溶剂前沿。在通风橱中挥干溶剂后，在紫外光照灯的254nm波长下观察暗斑，标出各斑点的位置、形状、并按比例描画图谱。找出各斑点中心点，用尺量出各斑点迁移距离和溶剂前沿移行距离，样品组分斑点的纵向宽度。

【数据记录与处理】

1. 薄层色谱数据记录

表11-1　磺胺类化合物的薄层色谱数据记录表

	溶剂前沿	SMZ 对照品	TMP 对照品	供试品	
				斑点1	斑点2
迁移距离 L（cm）					
纵向宽度 W（cm）	—	—	—		

2. 复方磺胺甲噁唑片的定性鉴定结果　根据比移值公式 $R_f = L / L_0$，分别计算 SMZ 和 TMP 对照品的比移值，样品斑点1和样品斑点2的比移值。根据分离度计算公式 $R = 2(L_2 - L_1) / (W_1 + W_2)$ 计算出样品斑点1和斑点2的分离度。

表11-2　复方磺胺甲噁唑片的定性鉴定结果表

	SMZ 对照品	TMP 对照品	供试品	
			斑点1	斑点2
比移值 R_f				
分离度 R	—	—		

【讨论与指导】

1. 薄层色谱分离条件选择　待测组分在薄层色谱法中是否能实现分离，关键在于固定相和展开剂的选择。

在药物分析中，硅胶是薄层色谱法最为常用的固定相，常用的展开剂有石油醚、甲苯、卤代烃、醇等有机溶剂。硅胶表面硅醇基的极性吸附作用是硅胶薄层色谱固定相的主要作用机制，可以根据"相似相溶"原则来选择展开剂。

极性较小的物质（如黄酮类、萜类、β-甾醇等），主要展开剂可以按石油醚、环己烷、甲苯、二甲苯、苯和三氯甲烷的优先顺序选择，调节 R_f 的溶剂按乙酸乙酯、甲醇、丙酮和乙醇的优先顺序选择。

中等极性物质（蒽醌、香豆素，皂苷类物质等），采用中等极性的溶剂体系：由三氯甲烷和水基本两相组成，由甲醇、乙醇、乙酸乙酯等调节溶剂体系的极性。

极性物质（如含氮的有机化合物：盐酸小檗碱、麻黄碱等），一般采用由正丁醇和水组成的强极性溶剂体系，甲醇、乙醇和有机酸（或有机碱）调节溶剂体系的极性和pH。

2. 薄层色谱法的展开方式　根据样品分析需要，可以选用不同的展开形式。

（1）单次展开　用同一种展开剂向一个方向展开一次，这种方式在平面色谱中应用最为广泛。

（2）多次展开　当一次展开未达到满意分离时，可将薄层板干燥后，再次用相同的展开剂沿同一方向重复展开，直至分离满意，在薄层色谱法应用也较多。

（3）梯度展开　当混合物中组分性质差别较大，一种流动相不能有效分离时，可以采用不同溶剂依次展开不同距离，使得每种组分都有自己合适的色谱条件，实现有效分离。

（4）双向展开（二维展开）　在两个垂直的方向展开，将样品点在薄层板的一端，展开适当距离后，挥干溶剂，再将薄层板以原展开方向成90度的方向展开。此法多用于成分较多、性质比较接近的难分离组分的分离。

Experiment 11　Identification of Sulfamethoxazole and Trimethoprim in Compound Sulfamethoxazole Tablets by Thin Layer Chromatography

1. Experimental Purposes

1.1 To learn the operation and principle of thin layer chromatography.

1.2 To learn the concept of Rf value and resolution.

1.3 To learn the application of thin layer chromatography in pharmaceutical analysis.

2. Experimental principles

2.1 The characters of sulfamethoxazole and trimethoprim

Sulfamethoxazole (SMZ) is a common sulfonamide antibiotic and widely used in antibacterial and antiinflammatory. The standard of SMZ is white crystalline powder with the density of 1.462g/cm^3, melting point of $166 \sim 169 ℃$, boiling point of $482℃$ and refractive index of 1.66. It is almost insoluble in water, slightly soluble in ethanol and freely soluble in acetone, the dilute sodium hydroxide solution and the dilute acid solution.

Trimethoprim (TMP) is an antimicrobial agent with antimicrobial range similar to sulfonamides. It can obviously produce synergism by ten to dozens of times when combined with sulfonamides. The standard of TMP is white crystalline powder with melting point of $199 \sim 203℃$. It is almost insoluble in water, slightly soluble in chloroform, ethanol and acetone, and freely soluble in glacial acetic acid.

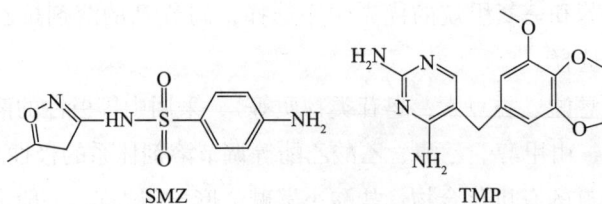

Fig. 11 – 1　The structures of SMZ and TMP

2. 2 The principle of thin layer chromatography

Thin layer chromatography (TLC) is a planar form of chromatography useful for qualitative analysis of pharmaceuticals by uniformly coating a smooth plate with a thin and adherent layer of finely divided adsorbents, then depositing samples onto the thin layer and developing sample by capillary action in mobile phase, finally identifying the component spots by comparing their positions with those of standards. Different sample components move up the plate at different rates to separate each other depending on the different interaction with the stationary phase and the mobile phase. The separation is characterized by the R_f value.

The R_f values are calculated by the following formula.

$$R_f = L / L_0$$

Where, L is the distance from the origin to the center of the component spot; L_0 is the distance from the starting line to the solvent front.

Sulfamethoxazole sample solution, SMZ and TMP reference solution are spotted onto a silica GF_{254} fluorescent thin layer plate and developed by trichloromethane – methanol – dimethylformamide (20 : 2 : 1) solution. SMZ and TMP in the sample will be separated by different absorption of silica and different solubility of mobile solution, and quench fluorescence of the thin layer plate to form dark spots. The R_f of the dark spots will be calculated and compared with those of reference substances on the same thin layer plate for the further identification.

The resolution (R) of SMZ and TMP is calculated by the following formula.

$$Resolution(R) = 2(L_2 - L_1)/(W_1 + W_2)$$

Where, L_1 and L_2 are the movement distances of two spots respectively; W_1 and W_2 are the longitudinal diameters of two spots respectively.

If $R = 1.0$, the two adjacent spots are basically separated.

3. Apparatus and Reagents

3. 1 Apparatus

Vertical chromatographic tank (20cm × 20cm); Glass plate (20cm × 5cm); Ultraviolet lamp (254nm); Capillary tubes (or micropipet); Small beaker (50ml); Horn spoon.

3. 2 Reagents

Compound sulfamethoxazole tablets (commercial products, each tablet containing 400mg SMZ and 80mg TMP); SMZ and TMP reference substance (national institute for the control of pharmaceutical and biological products); Trichloromethane – Methanol – Dimethylformamide solution (A. R,20 : 20 : 1,); Silica GF_{254}; Sodium Carboxymethylcellulose (CMC – Na) solution (0. 75g/ 100ml).

4. Experimental content

4. 1 Preparation of the reference solution

Accurately weigh 0. 2g of SMZ reference substance and 40mg of TMP reference substance, respectively. Then dissolve them with 10ml methanol and shake well before use.

4. 2 Preparation of the sample solution

Grind 10 tablets of compound sulfamethoxazole tablets into fine power, then take proper amount of fine powder (equivalent to about SMZ 0. 2g) and dissolve it with 10ml methanol and filter. The solution is filtered and the filtrate is used as the sample solution.

4. 3 Identification by TLC

a. Preparation of thin layer plate   Weigh silica GF$_{254}$ 6g with a balance and mix it with 17ml of CMC – Na aqueous solution (the ratio of silica to adhesives is about 1 : 3). Stir the mixture for 5minutes with the glass rod, then pour them onto the glass plates and spread them to the whole board by shaking and tilting the plates for several minutes until a uniform thickness of thin layer is obtained. Dry the plates in a well – ventilated place for days, then activate them at 110℃ for 1h and then store them in a desiccator.

b. Spotting   Draw a thin pencil line at about 2. 0cm from the bottom of the thin layer plate. Spot 5μl (about 1cm of the capillary tube) of SMZ reference solution, TMP reference solution and sulfonamide sample solution respectively on the thin plate by dot capillary with diameter no more than 3mm.

c. Developing   Pour 18ml (or an appropriate amount) of developing solvent into one side of the double – channel chromatographic tank to a depth of about 1cm, and place the plate into the other side of the chromatographic tank. Seal the tank and saturate the plate for 10 ~ 15minutes. After the saturation, transfer the plate into the developing solvent with its spotted end dipping in the developing solvent about 0. 3 ~ 0. 5cm deep and start developing. When the solvent front reaches approximately 10cm from the bottom of the plate, withdraw out the plate and draw another pencil line at this point immediately. The plate should be dried immediately.

d. Spot determination and data acquisition   After evaporation of the solvent, examine and mark the shape and position of the spots with a pencil under ultraviolet lamp at 254nm. Measure the distances travelled by each spot and the solvent and the longitudinal widths of the sample component spots to calculate the R_f and R.

5. Data record and processing

5. 1 Records of TLC

Table 11 – 1   Record of TLC

	Thesolvent front	SMZ reference	TMP reference	Sample	
				spot 1	spot 2
Movement distance (L, cm)					
Longitudinal width (W, cm)	—	—	—		

5. 2 Qualitative identification results of compound sulfamethoxazole

Calculate the R_f according to the following equation $R_f = L / L_0$. Calculate the R of the spot 1 and spot 2 according to the following equation $R = 2 (L_2 - L_1) / (W_1 + W_2)$.

Table 11 - 2　Qualitative identification results of compound sulfamethoxazole

	SMZ reference	TMP reference	Sample	
			spot 1	spot 2
Retention factor (R_f)				
Resolution (R)	—	—		

6. Discussion and guidance

6.1 The selection of TLC separation conditions

The appropriate stationary phase and mobile phase are keys for the TLC separation.

In pharmaceutical analysis, silica is widely used as the stationary phase in TLC and organic solvents such as petroleum ether, toluene, halogenated hydrocarbons and alcohols are commonly used as developers . The silanol group on the surface of silica has different polar adsorption on the components, which is the main mechanism of silica as the stationary phase in TLC. The developer is selected generally according its similarity with the measured components, which called "like dissolves like".

For small polarity substances such as flavonoids, terpenes and beta - sterols, the weak polar solvent system could be adopted. According to the priority order, these developers include petroleum ether, cyclohexane, toluene, xylene, benzene and chloroform, and the polarity regulators could be selected following the priority order of ethyl acetate, methanol, acetone and ethanol.

For medium polar substances such as anthraquinone, coumarin and saponins, a medium polar solvent system composed of chloroform and water could be chosen, with methanol, ethanol and ethyl acetate as polarity regulators.

For polar substances containing nitrogen such as berberine hydrochloride, andephedrine, strong polar solvent systems of n - butanol and water could be used and methanol, ethanol and organic acid (or organic base) regulate the polarity and the pH value of solvent systems.

6.2 The mode of developing in TLC

Different developing mode can be selected according to the requirement of the sample analysis.

a. Single developing is most widely used in thin layer chromatography, which means developing once in one direction with the same developer.

b. Multiple developing is also a common mode in thin layer chromatography. When the separation is unsatisfactory after the first developing, the thin layer plate can be dried and the same developing can be repeated with the same developer along the same direction until the satisfactory separation.

c. Gradient developing: when components with quite different nature in samples could not be separated by one kind of developer, different kinds of developer could be chosen to carry components forward for different distance, which can offer the optimal chromatographic conditions for each component in the sample for the separation.

d. Two - dimensional developing (Two - direction developing) means developing the sample in two vertical directions, which refers to dotting the sample at one corner of the thin layer, developing with a given solvent system for an appropriate distance, after drying the palte, turning the plate 90° and performing a further developing with another solvent system. This method is often used for the separation of mixtures with complex components and similar natures.

实验十二　气相色谱保留指数测定及其在定性分析中的应用

【实验目的】

1. 学习死时间的测定方法。
2. 学习保留指数的测定方法。
3. 学习保留指数在定性分析中的应用。

【实验原理】

1. 死时间的测定与计算　死时间（dead time，以t_M表示）：不保留物质从进样到柱后出现浓度最大值所需的时间，以秒（s）或者分钟（min）为单位表示。由于空气或甲烷等在固定液上都有一定的溶解度，可采用下式计算死时间更为准确：

$$t_M = \frac{t_{R(n+i)} \, t_{R(n-i)} - t_{R(n)}^2}{t_{R(n+i)} + t_{R(n-i)} - 2 \, t_{R(n)}} \tag{12-1}$$

式中，$t_{R(n+i)}$，$t_{R(n-i)}$，t_R分别为烷烃同系物中三个具有不同碳原子数的保留时间。

2. 调整保留时间　调整保留时间（adjusted retention time），以$t_R{}'$表示。保留时间扣除死时间后的保留值，其公式如下：

$$t_R{}' = t_R - t_M \tag{12-2}$$

在实验条件（温度、固定相等）一定时，调整保留时间只取决于组分的性质。因此，调整保留时间是色谱法定性的一个基本参数。

3. 保留指数　在一定色谱条件（固定相和操作条件）下，物质均有各自确定的保留值。因此，可利用保留值进行定性分析。常规保留值定性法存在标准品难得的不足。保留指数（retention index，以I表示），又称柯瓦兹指数（Kovats index），是使用最广泛，并被国际上公认的定性指标。它具有重现性好（精度可达 ± 0.1 指数单位）、标准物质统一、温度系数小等优点。它是将一个组分的保留行为换算成相当于含有 n 个碳正构烷烃的保留行为来描述，在色谱柱操作参数确定后，特定物质的 I 值应为一常数。所以，用 I 来对色谱峰定性就比单纯用常规保留值准确与可靠。

保留指数的计算统一用正构烷烃系列化合物作为标准物，规定在任何色谱条件下正构烷烃的保留指数均为所含碳数的 100 倍，即 $100N$（N 为正构烷烃的碳数）。恒温气相色谱中正构烷烃的流出以指数函数分布，其保留值的对数呈等间距间隔。在恒温条件下，选择一系列正构烷烃作为参考标准，被测物保留指数公式为：

$$I_x = 100n \frac{\lg t'_{R,x} - \lg t'_{R,N}}{\lg t'_{R,N+n} - \lg t'_{R,N}} + 100N \tag{12-3}$$

式中，I_x 为被测物的保留指数；$t'_{R,x}$ 为被测物的调整保留时间；$t'_{R,N}$，$t'_{R,N+n}$ 为 N、$N + n$

个碳原子正构烷烃的调整保留时间，n 常为1。

【仪器与试剂】

1. 仪器　气相色谱仪，FID 火焰离子化检测器，分析天平，容量瓶（10ml），微量注射器（1μl），气相进样针（1μl）。

2. 试剂　正构烷烃系列：$n-C_6H_{14}$，$n-C_8H_{18}$，$n-C_{10}H_{22}$；正构醇系列：$n-C_5H_{11}OH$，$n-C_6H_{13}OH$，$n-C_7H_{15}OH$ 及甲醇均为分析纯；高纯氮气，氢气，空气。

【实验内容】

1. 测试溶液的配制　精密移取三种正构烷烃各1μl至10ml 容量瓶，加甲醇溶解，并稀释至刻度，摇匀，作为正构烷烃混合液；精密移取三种正构醇各1μl至10ml 容量瓶，加甲醇溶解，并稀释至刻度，摇匀，作为正构醇混合液。

2. 色谱条件　Alltech ECONO EC-1 熔融石英毛细管柱（30m×0.32mm×1.0μm）或同类型色谱柱；柱温：90℃；载气：氮气；柱内流量：4ml/min；分流比：1：20；进样口温度：200℃；检测器温度：220℃；尾吹气：氮气；流速：燃气（H_2）流速30ml/min，助燃气（空气）流速300ml/min；进样量：1μl。

3. 进样分析　取1μl正构烷烃混合液或正构醇混合液注入气相色谱仪，测量至少三次计算保留时间平均值。

【数据记录与处理】

1. 色谱峰归属　在最佳色谱条件下，记录色谱图上各组分色谱峰保留时间。分析、判断色谱图中各峰的归属。

表 12-1　色谱峰归属

进样次数	正构烷烃			正构醇		
	t_R（min）	平均值	归属	t_R（min）	平均值	归属
第一次						
第二次						
第三次						

2. 计算死时间　选取3个链长增量相同的烷烃同系物保留时间，通过公式（12-1）计算死时间。

表12-2　烷烃保留时间与死时间

正构烷烃	进样次数	t_R（min）	平均值	t_M（min）
$n-C_6H_{14}$	1			
	2			
	3			
$n-C_8H_{16}$	1			
	2			
	3			
$n-C_{10}H_{18}$	1			
	2			
	3			

3. 正构醇保留指数的计算　通过公式（12-2）计算各分析物的调整保留时间，进一步通过公式（12-3）计算各正构醇的保留指数。

表12-3　正构醇的保留指数

正构烷烃				正构醇				I_x
C_n	t_R	t'_R	$\lg t'_R$	C_n	t_R	t'_R	$\lg t'_R$	正构醇

【实验指导与讨论】

1. 气相色谱中的保留规律　目前，气相色谱广泛使用的是毛细管柱。毛细管柱气相色谱中样品出峰顺序，主要依据色谱柱固定相类型和待测物特性。气相毛细管柱固定相通常可分为非极性柱、弱极性柱、中极性柱和强极性柱等。对于非极性柱，出峰顺序主要取决于待测物沸点。沸点低，出峰快而早；沸点高，出峰慢而晚。而在强极性柱里还受到样品极性影响，极性越大的物质出峰越慢。总之，无论用何种毛细管柱，沸点是影响色谱出峰顺序决定性因素，其次再考虑极性等其他因素。

2. 色谱定性的方法　目前药物色谱定性的常用方法主要有：①色谱定性分析最简便的方法是保留时间定性法；②相对保留时间和相对保留值；③保留指数定性。保留指数定性主要采用以下两种方式。

（1）一种是利用保留指数文献值参考定性　文献中大量已报导保留指数数值作为参考，通过使用与文献中相同的色谱条件测得未知物的保留指数，对照与文献值研判未知物的组成。

（2）另外一种是利用保留指数温度效应定性　各种物质保留指数随温度变化率是显著不同的，例如，不同烃类的保留指数随温度变化率大小的次序为：芳香烃 > 环烷烃 > 三取代烃 > 二取代烃和一取代烃。因此，利用这种规律可以进行未知物定性分析。

3. 保留指数定性的优点 在 GC 中，保留指数只与固定相类别和色谱柱温有关，所以保留指数定性比保留时间和相对保留值定性更可靠、更准确。保留指数与相对保留值比较而言，还具有标准物统一的特点。它采用正构烷烃作标准物，使被测化合物与标准物质之间尽可能在保留值上接近，这样会使保留指数值的计算更为准确；保留指数与化合物结构的相关性强于其它保留值，因而它具有判别化合物结构的功能；保留指数是对数值，同系物的保留指数值与化合物碳数成直线关系；目前文献中已有大量气相色谱保留指数的数据可供查阅与比对。

Experiment 12　Determination of Retention Index of Gas Chromatography and its Application in Qualitative Analysis

1. Experimental Purposes

1. 1 To learn the calculation method of the dead time.

1. 2 To learn the determination method of the retention index.

1. 3 To learn the application of retention index in qualitative analysis.

2. Experimental principles

2. 1 Calculation of dead time

Dead time (Expressed in t_M) : The time required for the maximum concentration of non – retained substances to occur from the injector to post – column, represented in seconds (s) or minutes (min). Because air or methane has a certain solubility in stationary liquid, the following formula can be used to calculate the dead time more accurately：

$$t_M = \frac{t_{R(n+i)}\, t_{R(n-i)} - t_{R(n)}^2}{t_{R(n+i)} + t_{R(n-i)} - 2\, t_{R(n)}} \qquad (12-1)$$

In formula, $t_{R(n+i)}$, $t_{R(n-i)}$, t_R are the retention times of three alkanes with different carbon atom numbers in the homologues.

2. 2 Adjusted retention time

Adjusted retention time (Expressed in t'_R), the retention time after deducting the dead time is formulated as follows：

$$t'_R = t_R - t_M \qquad (12-2)$$

When the experimental conditions (temperature, stationary equivalence) are constant, the adjusted retention time only depends on the properties of components. Therefore, the adjusted retention time is a basic parameter for the qualitative analysis in chromatography.

2. 3 Retention index

Under the fixed chromatographic conditions (stationary phase and operating condition), the retention values of compounds are constant. Therefore, the retention value can be used for the qualitative analysis but suffer from the lack of reference substances. Retention index (I), also known as

Kovats index, is the most widely used and internationally recognized qualitative indicator, which has the advantages of good reproducibility (accuracy up to 0.1 exponential units), unification of standard substances and small temperature coefficient. The Kovats index describes the retention behavior of a component by converting it into the retention behavior of n – alkanes. Under the fixed parameters of the chromatographic column, the I value of the analyte is constant. Therefore, the identification of the chromatographic peak by I value is much more reliable than the relative retention value.

The retention index is calculated by using n – alkanes as standard materials. It is stipulated that the retention index of n – alkanes under any chromatographic conditions is 100 times of the number of carbon contained, i. e. 100 N (N is the number of carbon of n – alkanes). The outflow of normal alkanes in isothermal gas chromatography is distributed by exponential function, so the logarithm of its retention value is equidistant. Under the constant temperature, a series of n – alkanes are used as reference standards. The retention index formula of the tested compound is as follows:

$$I_x = 100n \frac{\lg t'_{R,x} - \lg t'_{R,N}}{\lg t'_{R,N+n} - \lg t'_{R,N}} + 100N \qquad (12-3)$$

Where, I_x: Retention index of measured compound; $t'_{R,x}$: Adjustment retention time of measured compound; $t'_{R,N}$, $t'_{R,N+n}$: The adjusted retention time of n – alkanes with N and $N+n$ carbon atoms, usually $n = 1$.

3. Apparatus and Reagents

3.1 Apparatus

Gas chromatography system; Flame ionization detector (FID); Analytical balance; Volumetric flask (10ml); Microsyringe (1μl); Manual injection syringe for GC (1μl).

3.2 Reagents

N – alkanes series ($n - C_6H_{14}$, $n - C_8H_{18}$, $n - C_{10}H_{22}$); N – alcohols series ($n - C_5H_{11}OH$, $n - C_6H_{13}OH$, $n - C_7H_{15}OH$) and methanol are all analytical reagent (AR); High purity nitrogen; Hydrogen; Air.

4. Experimental contents

4.1 Preparation of test solutions

Accurately pipette 1μl of each n – alkane to a 10ml volumetric flask, then dissolve them with methanol to the mark and shake well as the normal alkane mixed solution.

Accurately pipette 1μl of each n – alcohol to a 10ml volumetric flask, then dissolve them with methyl alcohol to the mark and shake well as the normal alcohol mixed solution.

4.2 Setting of gas chromatography conditions

Alltech ECONO EC – 1 fused silica capillary column (30m × 0.32mm × 1.0μm) or similar columns is used as the stationary phase. The column temperature is 90℃. The carrier gas is nitrogen. The column flow is about 4ml/min and the split ratio is 1 ∶ 20. The inlet temperature and hydrogen flame detector temperature are 200℃ and 220℃, respectively. The tail blowing gas is nitrogen. The 30ml/min of hydrogen is used as the burning gas. Air as assistant gas is set at 300ml/min. The volume of injection is $1\mu l$.

4. 3 Sample analysis

Inject $1\mu l$ of the normal alkane mixed solution or normal alcohol mixed solution into the gas chromatography system at least three times to measure the average retention time.

5. Data record and processing

5. 1 Assignment of chromatographic peaks

Under the optimal chromatographic conditions, the retention time of chromatographic peaks of each component in the chromatogram was recorded and assigned.

Table 12 - 1　Assignment of chromatographic peaks

Number of injection	n - alkane			n - alcohol		
	t_R (min)	Average value	Assignment	t_R (min)	Average value	Assignment
The first injection						
The second injection						
The third injection						

5. 2 Calculation of the dead time

The dead time can be calculated from the retention time of alkane homologues according to the formula $(2-1)$.

Table 12 - 2　Calculation of dead time

N - alkanes	Number of injection	t_R (min)	Average value	t_M (min)
$n - C_6H_{14}$	1			
	2			
	3			
$n - C_8H_{16}$	1			
	2			
	3			
$n - C_{10}H_{18}$	1			
	2			
	3			

5. 3 The retention index of n - alcohols

Calculate the adjusted retention time of each analyte by the formula $(2-2)$ and further calculate the retention index of each n – alcohol by the formula （2 – 3）.

Table 12 – 3　Retention index of n – alcohols

n – alkanes				n – alcohols				I_x
C_n	t_R	t'_R	lg t'_R	C_n	t_R	t'_R	lg t'_R	n – alcohols

6. Discussion and guidance

6. 1 The retention order of analytes in GC

Capillary column is widely used in gas chromatography. The type of stationary phase and the characters of analyte are two main factors on the retention order in GC. Generally, the stationary phase of capillary column is divided into non – polar column, weak polar column, neutral column and strong polar column. For non – polar column, the retention order is mainly depend on the boiling point of analytes. The higher boiling point analyte has the stronger retention. For the strong polarity column, the polarity of the sample also affects the retention order. The analyte with larger polarity has the stronger retention. No matter what kind of capillary column is used, the boiling point of analyte is the decisive factor affecting the retention order. Secondly, other factors such as polarity of analyte should be considered.

6. 2 Qualitative methods in chromatography

Qualitative analysis by the retention time of analyte is the simplest method in chromatography. Other qualitative methods include relative retention time, relative retention value and retention index. Two ways are used for the application of the retention index in qualitative analysis in chromatography.

The first way is the comparison of retention index with the reported value: a large number of retention index values have been reported in the literature as reference. Therefore, the retention index of unknown compound can be measured by using the same chromatographic conditions as in the literature and it can be identified by comparing the retention index values with those in the literature.

The second way is identification based on the temperature effect of retention index. The change rate of retention index of different substances with temperature is significantly different. For example, the order of the change rate of retention index of different hydrocarbons with temperature is: aromatic hydrocarbon > naphthenic hydrocarbon > trisubstituted hydrocarbon > disubstituted hydrocarbon and one substituted hydrocarbon. Therefore, this rule can be used for the qualitative analysis for the unknown compound.

6. 3 The advantage of retention index for the qualitative analysis

In GC, the retention index of analyte only depends on the type of stationary phase and column temperature. Therefore, the qualitative analysis by the relative retention value is more reliable and accurate than that by the retention time. When compared with the relative retention value, the advantage of retention index is the unification of standard substances. The retention index uses all n-alkanes as standard substances, so that the retention values between the tested compounds and the standard substances are as close as possible, which makes its calculation more accurate. Retention index has a stronger correlation with the structure of compounds than other retention values, so it has the function of discriminating the structure of compounds. The retention index is alogarithmic value, and the *I* value of a group of homologues is linear with the carbon number of the compounds. At present, a large number of compounds have been reported their retention index values in gas chromatography and it is convenient for the comparison with the unknown compound.

实验十三　高效液相色谱法鉴别尿样中的巴比妥类药物

【实验目的】

1. 学习高效液相色谱法的定性鉴别原理。
2. 学习滥用药物鉴别的意义。
3. 学习处理尿样的方法。

【实验原理】

1. 滥用药物　在当前社会中，药品滥用成为危害社会稳定的一个严重隐患，巴比妥类药物的滥用就是其中的一个主要部分。巴比妥类药物为临床上广泛应用的镇静催眠药，其临床安全和合理用药有明确管制，且易被滥用，对于巴比妥类药物中毒患者或者滥用患者进行快速鉴别分析，对于临床抢救具有重要意义。巴比妥类药物口服易从碱性肠液吸收，入血后迅速分布全身组织和体液中。巴比妥类药物在体内主要有两种消除方式。一种经肝脏氧化，另一种以原形由肾脏排泄，例如苯巴比妥有48%左右在肝脏氧化，15%～20%以原形由尿液排出。因此，可以利用尿液来鉴别患者滥用的巴比妥类药物的种类。

2. 巴比妥类药物的性质　巴比妥类药物均为巴比妥酸的衍生物，为环状酰脲类镇静催眠药，其基本结构通式如下：

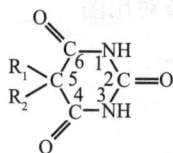

图 13-1　巴比妥类药物

表 13-1　常见巴比妥类药物的化学结构

药物	R_1	R_2
巴比妥	—C_2H_5	—C_2H_5
苯巴比妥	—C_2H_5	—C_6H_5
司可巴比妥	—$CH_2CH=CH_2$	—$CH(CH_3)(CH_2)_2CH_3$
戊巴比妥	—C_2H_5	—$CH(CH_3)(CH_2)_2CH_3$
异戊巴比妥	—C_2H_5	—$CH_2CH_2CH(CH_3)_2$
硫喷妥钠	—C_2H_5	—C_2H_5

扫码"学一学"

扫码"看一看"

【仪器与试剂】

1. 仪器　高效液相色谱仪，紫外检测器，分析天平，高速离心机，超声波清洗器，微量移液器（1000μl、200μl），涡旋混合振荡器，量瓶（100ml、10ml），量筒（500ml），离心管（5ml、1.5ml），吸液头（1000μl、100μl），移液管（5ml，1ml）。

2. 试剂　巴比妥对照品（中国食品药品检定研究院），苯巴比妥对照品（中国食品药品检定研究院），异戊巴比妥对照品（中国食品药品检定研究院）；空白尿液、待测尿液；甲醇为色谱纯试剂，水为去离子水。

【实验内容】

1. 对照品溶液的配制　分别精密称取三种巴比妥类对照品约1mg，分别置10ml量瓶中，加甲醇溶解并稀释制成每1ml含100μg的对照品溶液，4℃冷藏备用。

2. 尿液样品的处理　分别吸取空白尿液和待测尿液200μl，置1.5ml EP管中，加入乙腈0.2ml，涡旋3分钟，12000 rpm离心5分钟，精密吸取上层溶液，分别作为空白尿液样品和待测尿液样品。

3. 色谱条件设置　色谱柱：Lichrospher ODS（250mm×4.6mm×5μm）或同类色谱柱；流动相：甲醇：水（70：30）；流速1.0ml/min；检测波长254nm；温度：室温；进样量：20μl。

4. 定性鉴别　精密吸取对照品溶液各20μl，分别注入高效液相色谱仪，记录色谱图；精密吸取空白尿液样品和待测尿液样品各20μl，分别注入高效液相色谱仪，记录色谱图。

【数据记录与处理】

1. 对照品溶液和待测尿液样品的保留时间测定记录

表13－1　保留时间测定记录

样品	巴比妥对照品	苯巴比妥对照品	异戊巴比妥对照品	待测尿液样品
t_R（min）				
峰面积				

2. 空白尿样和待测尿液样品的色谱对比图

3. 待测尿液样品与对照品溶液的色谱对比图

【讨论与指导】

1. 高效液相色谱的鉴定方法　利用高效液相色谱的主要保留时间来对化合物进行定性鉴别的方法具有一定的局限性，存在假阳性的可能，证据不够充分；如果使用DAD检测器，结合待测药物的紫外光谱图谱比对，可以进一步提升结果的可靠性。如果实验室条件允许，使用液质联用或者气质联用技术，通过与对照品比对色谱保留时间，母离子分子量和碎片离子分子量一致，可获得最终的铁证。

2. 尿液样品的前处理方法 尿液的主要成分是水、含氮化合物（大部分是尿素）及盐类，若肾脏的功能正常，在尿液中仅存在极少量的蛋白，但是当肾脏与尿管出现障碍时就会变成蛋白尿。因此尿液不能直接进入色谱系统进行分析，仍然要根据尿液中的药物浓度及分析方法的灵敏度选择样品前处理方法。本实验中需快速鉴别巴比妥类药物，繁琐的液液提取法并不适合，因此采用一倍体积的乙腈直接沉淀处理尿液，既可除去尿液中的微量蛋白，又简单快捷，此外，还可避免进样时的"溶剂效应"。如果有机溶剂沉淀法灵敏度不够，可考虑液液提取法或者固相萃取法，并增大尿液的取用量，达到"富集"待分析物，提高灵敏度的目的；或者考虑更换更灵敏的检测仪器，比如液质联用。

Experiment 13　Identification of Barbiturates in Urine Samples by HPLC

1. Experimental Purposes

1. 1 To learn the principle of HPLC identification.

1. 2 To learn the importance for the identification of drug abuse.

1. 3 To learn the method for the preparation of urine samples.

2. Experimental principles

2. 1 Drug abuse

In the current society, drug abuse has become a serious trouble to social stability, and the abuse of barbiturates is a major part of it. As the asedativehypnotic drug, barbiturates are widely used in clinical practice. Its clinical usage about safety are clearly regulated, and the drugs are easily abused. Rapid identification and analysis of barbiturate poisoning or abuse is important for patient rescue.

Barbiturates are easily absorbed in alkaline intestinal fluids and are rapidly distributed in systemic tissues and body fluids after released into blood. There are two ways to eliminate barbiturates in the body. One is oxidized by the liver, and the other is excreted by the kidney in its original form. For example, about 48% of phenobarbital is oxidized in the liver, and 15% to 20% is directly excreted by urine. Therefore, urine can be used to identify the type of barbiturates in the patients.

2. 2 The characters of barbiturates

Barbiturates are derivatives of barbituric acid, which are cyclic ureide sedative – hypnotics. The graphic formula is as follows:

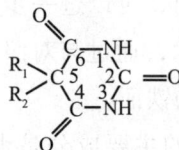

Fig. 13 – 1   Barbiturates

Table 13 – 1   Chemical structure of barbiturates

Drug	R_1	R_2
Barbital	$-C_2H_5$	$-C_2H_5$
Phenobarbital	$-C_2H_5$	$-C_6H_5$
Secobarbital	$-CH_2CH=CH_2$	$-CH(CH_3)(CH_2)_2CH_3$
Pentobarbital	$-C_2H_5$	$-CH(CH_3)(CH_2)_2CH_3$
Amobarbital	$-C_2H_5$	$-CH_2CH_2CH(CH_3)_2$
Thiopental sodium	$-C_2H_5$	$-C_2H_5$

3. Apparatus and Reagents

3. 1 Apparatus

High performance liquid chromatography system with UV Detector; Analytical balance; High speed centrifuge; Ultrasonic cleaning instrument; Micropipettor ($1000\mu l$, $200\mu l$); Vortex mixer; Volumetric flask ($100ml$, $10ml$), Graduated cylinder ($500ml$); Centrifuge tube ($5ml$, $1.5ml$); Pipette tips ($1000\mu l$, $100\mu l$), Transfer pipette ($5ml$, $1ml$).

3. 2 Reagents

Barbiturate reference substance, phenobarbital reference substance and amobarbital reference substance (National institute for the control of pharmaceutical and biological products); Blank urine and unknown urine; Methanol is HPLC grade reagent; Water is deionized.

4. Experimental contents

4. 1 Preparation of reference solutions

Weigh about 1mg each of the barbiturate reference substances to a 10ml volumetric flask respectioely, dissolve and dilute them with methanol to the mark to prepare $100\mu g/ml$ reference solutions. Reference solutions are all stored at 4℃ for the use.

4. 2 Preparation of urine samples

Separately pipette $200\mu l$ of blank urine and unknown urine in a 1.5ml EP tube, add 0.2ml of acetonitrile, vortex for 3min and centrifuge at 12000 rpm for 5min. The supernatants are recorded as the blank urine sample and the unknown urine sample, respectively.

4. 3 Chromatographic conditions

Lichrospher ODS ($250mm \times 4.6mm \times 5\mu m$) or similar chromatographic column is used as the stationary phase. The mobile phase is a mixture of methanol and water ($v/v = 70 : 30$). The flow rate is $1.0ml/min$ and the column temperature is room temperature. The detection wavelength is

254nm and the injection volume is 20μl.

4. 4 Qualitative identification

Inject 20μl of each reference solution into the HPLC system to obtain the chromatograms. Then inject 20μl of the blank urine sample and the unknown urine sample into the HPLC system to obtain the chromatograms, respectively.

5. Data record and processing

5. 1 Record for the t_R of reference solutions and the unknown urine sample

Table 13 – 2　Record for the t_R

Sample	Barbiturate reference solution	Phenobarbital reference solution	Amobarbital reference solution	Urine sample
t_R (min)				
Area				

5. 2 The chromatograms of the blank urine sample and the unknown urine sample

5. 3 The chromatograms of the unknown urine sample and the respective reference solution

6. Discussion and guidance

6. 1 The HPLC identification methods

It has potential false positives to identify compounds only by retention time, and the result is inaccurate. DAD detector combines with the UV spectrum of the drug can improve the reliability of the results. If the experimental conditions are available, LC/MS or GC/MS can be employed in this experiment, through which reliable results can be obtained by comparing the molecular weight of the parent ion and the fragment ion at t_R of the reference with the sample.

6. 2 The preparation methods of urine samples

Urine is mainly composed of water, nitrogenous compounds (mostly urea) and salts. There is very little protein in normal urine, but it becomes proteinuria when the kidneys or ureters are diseased. Therefore, urine sample cannot be analyzed directly by HPLC. Pretreatment method should be established based on the drug concentration in the urine and the sensitivity of the analytical method. It is necessary to quickly identify barbiturates in this experiment. The liquid – liquid extraction method is too cumbersome. Pretreating urine with acetonitrile can precipitate proteins and avoid the "solvent effect", which is simple and rapid. It can enrich the analytes and improve sensitivity by using liquid – liquid extraction or solid – phase extraction while increasing the amount of urine. LC/MS can also improve sensitivity.

扫码"练一练"

第四章 色谱技术在体内药物分析中的应用

Chapter 4 Application of Chromatographic techniques in Biopharmaceutical Analysis

实验十四 有机溶剂沉淀法测定血浆中茶碱的浓度

【实验目的】

1. 学习有机溶剂沉淀法处理血浆的方法。
2. 学习标准曲线的制备和"模拟血浆浓度"的概念。
3. 学习高效液相色谱测定血浆中药物含量的方法。

【实验原理】

1. 药物简介　茶碱，即 1，3 - 二甲基 - 3，7 - 二氢 - 1H - 嘌呤 - 2，6 - 二酮一水合物，分子式为 $C_7H_8N_4O_2 \cdot H_2O$，分子量为 198.18。白色结晶性粉末，易溶于氢氧化钾溶液或氨溶液，微溶于乙醇或三氯甲烷，在乙醚中几乎不溶。茶碱用于治疗支气管哮喘及其他呼吸不正常的疾病，近代医学用于早产婴儿的窒息。茶碱的治疗血药浓度较窄（5 ~ 20μg/ml），血药浓度高于 25μg/ml 时，常出现中毒症状。而且服用同剂量茶碱的病人之间的治疗效果有显著差异，这与血药浓度有关，因此需进行临床用药监护。血浆中茶碱可以用沉淀法进行样品前处理，也可用有机溶剂提取、挥干，以流动相复溶后，以 HPLC 分离，以内标法进行定量。内标可选择咖啡因，分子式为 $C_8H_{10}N_4O_2$，分子量为 194.19，与茶碱结构近似，化学性质和色谱保留行为也近似。

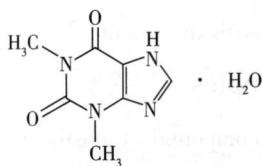

茶碱（Theophylline，THP）　　　咖啡因（Caffine）（内标，CAF）

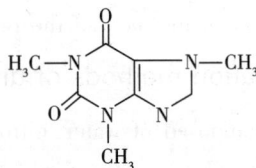

图 14 - 1　茶碱和咖啡因的结构

2. 生物样本测定中的标准曲线法　由于生物体内药物浓度范围较宽，因此生物样本测定中一般采用标准曲线法。生物样本测定中所用的标准曲线的判断标准，除了要求相关系数 $r \geqslant 0.99$，还应该用回归得到的线性方程来计算标准曲线中各个浓度点的准确度，最低浓度点准确度要求在 80% ~ 120%，其余浓度点的准确度要求在 85% ~ 115%。如果直接用不引入权重系数的普通最小二乘法求算回归方程，通常会导致低浓度区域计算值相对误差过大，标准曲线的准确度常常不合格，为了克服这一局限性，在实际工作中通常采用加权最小二乘法，引入权重系数赋予低浓度点更大的权重，兼顾考虑低中高浓度点的准确度。

3. 有机溶剂沉淀法 有机溶剂沉淀法是一种常用的去除血浆中蛋白质的方法，其原理是使蛋白质的分子内及分子间的氢键发生变化而使蛋白质凝聚。常用有机溶剂有乙腈和甲醇，有机溶剂与血浆或血清按体积比为（1～3）：1 混合后高速（12000 转/分钟）离心 1～2 分钟分离，取上清液作为分析样品。有机溶剂沉淀处理血浆样本简单快捷，但存在"稀释"效应，要求待测药物浓度较高，处理得到的进样溶液内源性物质残留较多，需要优化色谱条件，使待测物避开内源性物质的干扰。

【仪器与试剂】

1. 仪器 高效液相色谱仪，紫外检测器，微量注射器（10μl），分析天平，离心机，超声波清洗器，微量移液器（1000μl、200μl），涡旋混合振荡器，量瓶（100ml、10ml），量筒（500ml），离心管（5ml、1.5ml），吸液头（1000μl、100μl），移液管（5ml、1ml）。

2. 试剂 茶碱对照品（中国食品药品检定研究院），咖啡因对照品（中国食品药品检定研究院）；空白血浆、含药待测血浆；乙腈为分析纯试剂，甲醇为色谱纯试剂，水为去离子水。

【实验内容】

1. 对照品溶液的制备

（1）茶碱对照品溶液 精密称取茶碱对照品 100mg，置 100ml 量瓶中，用水溶解，并稀释制成每 1ml 含 1000μg 的对照品储备液，精密量取茶碱对照品储备液适量，用水稀释制成浓度分别为 50.0、125.0、250.0、500.0 和 1000.0μg/ml 的茶碱标准系列溶液，4℃冷藏。

（2）咖啡因内标溶液 精密称取咖啡因对照品 10mg，置 100ml 量瓶中，用甲醇溶解，并定量稀释制成每 1ml 含 100μg 的储备溶液；精密量取该溶液 1.0ml 置 100ml 量瓶中，用甲醇稀释至刻度配成 1μg/ml 的标准溶液，4℃冷藏。

2. 血浆样品处理方法 取冷冻的血浆样品，在 37℃ 水浴下解冻，精密吸取 250μl，置 1.5ml EP 管中，精密加入内标溶液 25μl，精密加入空白甲醇溶液 25μl（如果制备标准曲线，替换为 25μl 相应浓度的系列对照品溶液），涡旋 10 秒混匀，精密加入乙腈 0.5ml，涡旋混合 2 分钟，12000 rpm 离心 5 分钟，分取上清液 100μl，置于另一干燥 EP 管中，精密加入 100μl 流动相，涡旋 10 秒混匀，取 20μl 进样。

3. 特异性 按"血浆样品处理"项下的方法，制备空白血浆（不含茶碱和内标）、茶碱样品（不含内标，标准曲线中间浓度点）和内标样品（不含茶碱）3 种样品，进样 20μl，记录色谱图。通过色谱图比对，判断空白血浆对茶碱和内标的出峰位置有无内源性干扰，确定待测组分茶碱和内标的保留时间。

4. 标准曲线的制备 取空白血浆 250μl，分别置 2ml EP 管中，精密加入 50.0、125.0、250.0、500.0 和 1000.0μg/ml 的茶碱标准系列溶液各 25μl，按"血浆样品处理"项下同法处理，进样 20μl，记录色谱图。以茶碱血浆浓度为横坐标，茶碱与内标的峰面积比值为纵坐标，用最小二乘法进行回归运算，求得的直线回归方程即为标准曲线。

5. 色谱条件设置 色谱柱：Lichrospher ODS（250mm×4.6mm×5μm）或同类色谱柱；

流动相：甲醇：水（50：50）；流速 1.0ml/min；检测波长 254nm；温度：室温；进样量：20μl。

6. 样品测定 取"特异性"项下样品（空白血浆样品、仅含茶碱的血浆样品和仅含内标的血浆样品），在茶碱和内标出峰位置应无血浆内源性干扰，茶碱与内标的分离度应符合规定，理论板数按茶碱峰计算应不低于 3000。取"标准曲线"项下系列浓度血浆样品和待测未知样品分别处理、测定，记录色谱图。将茶碱与内标的峰面积比值代入标准曲线，按内标法求算未知样品的茶碱血药浓度。

【数据记录与处理】

1. 样品制备记录表和实验数据记录表

表 14 – 1　样品制备记录表

实验内容	特异性			标准曲线					未知样品
样品标记	0	0 + IS	0 + THP	1	2	3	4	5	X
空白血浆	√	√	√	√	√	√	√	√	待测血浆
茶碱	×	×	√	√	√	√	√	√	空白甲醇
内标	×	√	×	√	√	√	√	√	√

√：添加　×：不加

表 14 – 2　实验数据记录表

NO.	模拟 $C_{(THP)}$	THP		CAF		A_{THP}/A_{CAF}
		t_R	峰面积 A	t_R	峰面积 A	
空白						
空白 + 内标						
空白 + 茶碱						
1						
2						
3						
4						
5						
未知样品						

2. 特异性样品色谱图

3. 标准曲线回归方程的评价

表 14 – 3　标准曲线回归方程的评价

	模拟 $C_{(THP)}$	$a_{(THP/CAF)}$	计算 $C_{(THP)}$	准确度（%）
1				
2				
3				
4				
5				
回归方程				

4. 利用标准曲线回归方程计算未知样本中的药物浓度

【讨论与指导】

1. 理解特异性实验的目的 方法的特异性，又称专属性或专一性，系指当有内源性物质存在时，方法准确测定待测物质的能力。本实验中需要确定茶碱和内标的色谱峰位置；判断空白血浆中内源性物质是否干扰茶碱和内标的色谱峰。

2. "模拟血药浓度"的含义 注意标准曲线回归时应采用"模拟血药浓度"与仪器响应值进行回归，而不是进样时的处理后溶液中的药物浓度，也不是对照品溶液的浓度。在制备标准曲线时在规定体积的空白血浆中加入了一定体积的对照品溶液，为了消除体积引起的误差，所以在处理未知样品时需要补足相同体积的空白甲醇。

3. 样品处理 最后一步用流动性稀释一倍，可避免进样时的"溶剂效应"，获得满意的色谱峰形。

4. 移液器的使用

（1）在调节量程时，如果从小体积调为大体积时，可先旋转刻度旋钮至较大体积的刻度，再回调至设定体积，这样可以保证量取的最高精确度。不可将按钮旋出最大量程，否则会卡住内部机械装置损坏移液枪。

（2）装配枪头时应将移液枪（器）垂直插入枪头中，稍微用力左右微微转动即可使其紧密结合。

（3）吸取液体时，移液器保持竖直状态，将枪头插入液面下 2～3 毫米，在吸液之前，可以先吸放几次液体以润湿吸液嘴（尤其是要吸取黏稠或密度与水不同的液体时）。可采取两种移液方法：一是前进移液法，用大拇指将按钮按下至第一停点，然后慢慢松开按钮吸取液体回原点，接着将按钮按至第一停点排出液体，稍停片刻继续按按钮至第二停点吹出残余的液体，最后松开按钮。二是反向移液法。此法一般用于转移高黏液体、生物活性液体、易起泡液体或极微量的液体，其原理就是先吸入多于设置量程的液体，转移液体的时候不用吹出残余的液体。先按下按钮至第二停点，慢慢松开按钮至原点。接着将按钮按至第一停点排出设置好量程的液体，继续保持按住按钮位于第一停点（千万别再往下按），取下有残留液体的枪头，弃之。

（4）使用完毕，将其竖直挂在移液枪架上，当枪头里有液体时，切勿将移液器水平放置或倒置，以免液体倒流腐蚀活塞弹簧。

Experiment 14　Determination of Theophylline in Plasma by Organic Solvent Precipitation

1. Experimental Purposes

1.1 To learn the organic solvent precipitation method for plasma treatment.

1.2 To learn the calibration curve preparation and the concept of "simulated plasma concentration".

1.3 To learn the methods for the determination of drugs in plasma by HPLC.

2. Experimental principle

2. 1 The characters of Theophylline

Theophylline is $1,3$ – dimethyl – $3,7$ – dihydro – $1H$ – indole – $2,6$ – dione monohydrate with the molecular formula of $C_7H_8N_4O_2 \cdot H_2O$ and molecular weight of $198. 18$. It is white crystalline powder, freely soluble in potassium hydroxide solution or ammonia solution, slightly soluble in ethanol or chloroform and practically insoluble in ether. Theophylline is commonly used in medicine, such as the treatment of bronchial asthma and other abnormal respiratory diseases. Premature infant asphyxia is treated with theophylline in modern medicine. Its therapeutic index is very narrow($5 \sim 20\mu g/ml$) and toxic symptom often appears when blood concentrations of theophylline is higher than $25\mu g/ml$. Furthermore, there is significant difference in therapeutic effect among patients with the same dosage, which is related to blood concentration. So, theophylline should be monitored with care in clinical practice. Theophylline in plasma can be pretreated by precipitation or be extracted with organic solvent then volatilized and the residues are reconstituted in the mobile phase. The samples are separated and quantified with internal standard method of HPLC.

Caffeine is selected as the internal standard with molecular formula of $C_8H_{10}N_4O_2$ and molecular weight of $194. 19$. The structure of caffeine is close to theophylline and their chemical properties and chromatographic retention behaviors are similar.

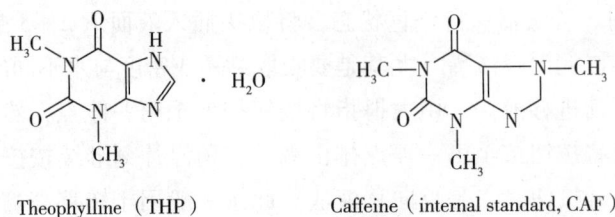

Theophylline （THP）   Caffeine（internal standard, CAF）

Fig. 14 – 1   The structure of Theophylline

2. 2 The calibration curve method in biopharmaceutical analysis

Because the concentrations of drugs in biological samples cover a wide range, the calibration curve method is often used for the determination of drugs in biopharma – ceutical analysis. For the calibration curve method in biopharmaceutical analysis, the correlation coefficient should be greater than $0. 99$ and the accuracy should be within $\pm 20\%$ at the lowest concentration level and within $\pm 15\%$ at all the other levels calculated by the regression method. The ordinary least squares method without weight coefficients is adopted to calculate regression equation. This method usually results in large relative error of the calculated value in low concentration region and unqualified accuracy of the calibration curve. In order to overcome this limitation, the weighted least squares method is applied practical work. A greater weight is given to low concentration points to ensure the accuracy of each concentration points.

2. 3 Organic solvent precipitation

Organic solvent precipitation is a commonly used method to remove protein from plasma. Its principle is to change the hydrogen bonds within and between molecules of protein to coagulate proteins. Commonly used organic solvents include acetonitrile and methanol. Organic solvents are mixed with plasma or serum at a volume ratio of 1 : 1 to 3 : 1, and then centrifuged at a high speed (12000 rpm) for 1 – 2minutes. The supernatant is taken as the analytical sample. Organic solvent precipitation is a simple and rapid method to prepare plasma sample, but there is a "dilution effect" and more endogenous substances will remain in the injection solution. Therefore, it requires a higher concentration of the test sample and chromatographic conditions optimization to avoid the interference of endogenous substances.

3. Apparatus and Reagents

3. 1 Apparatus

High performance liquid chromatography system with UV Detector; Microliter syringe (10μl); Analytical balance; Centrifuge; Ultrasonic cleaning instrument; Vortex mixer; Micropipettor (1000μl, 200μl); Volumetric flask (100ml, 10ml); Graduated cylinder (500ml); Centrifuge tubes (5ml, 1. 5ml); Pipet tips (1000μl, 100μl); Transfer pipette (5ml, 1ml).

3. 2 Reagents

Theophylline reference substance (National institute for the control of pharmaceutical and biological products); Caffeine reference substance (National institute for the control of pharmaceutical and biological products); Blank plasma; Acetonitrile is analytical reagent; Methanol is HPLC grade reagent; Water is deionized.

4. Experimental contents

4. 1 Preparation of the standard solution

Standard solution of theophylline: Accurately weigh 100mg of theophylline reference substance to a 100ml volumetric flask, dissolve and diluent with water to volume to prepare a stock solution of theophylline (1000μg/ml). The stock solution is further diluted with water to obtain standard solutions of 50. 0, 125. 0, 250. 0, 500. 0 and 1000. 0μg/ml respectively. The stock and standard solutions are all stored at 4℃ in the refrigerator.

Standard solution of caffeine: Accurately weigh 10mg of caffeine reference substance to 100ml volumetric flask, dissolve with methanol to make a stock solution of caffeine (100μg/ml). The stock solution is further diluted with methanol to obtain standard solution of 1. 0μg/ml. Keep at 4℃ for further use.

4. 2 Preparation of plasma samples

Thaw the frozen plasma samples in 37℃ water bath. Precisely pipette 250μl of it to a 1. 5ml EP tube, add 25μl of the internal standard solution and 25μl of blank methanol solution (if the calibration curve is prepared, replace with 25μl of standard solution of corresponding concentration). Then vortex the mixture for 10s, add 0. 5ml of acetonitrile precisely, vortex for 2min to mix well. Centrifuge it at 12000rpm for 5min. Transfer 100μl of the supernate to another dry EP tube. Precisely add 100μl of mobile phase, vortex for 10s to mix well, then inject 20μl into the chromatography system.

4. 3 Specificity

Prepare blank plasma (without theophylline and internal standard), theophylline sample (without internal standard, corresponding to the intermediate concentration of calibration curve) and internal standard sample (without theophylline) with reference to '4.2 Preparation of plasma samples' respectively. Inject 20μl into the chromatography system and record the chromatogram. The endogenous interference of blank plasma at the position of theophylline and the internal standard is judged by comparing chromatogram. The retention time of theophylline and the internal standard are determined meanwhile.

4.4 Preparation of calibration curve

To each of 250μl of blank plasma in 2ml EP tubes, add 25μl of a series of theophylline standard solution of 50.0, 125.0, 250.0, 500.0 and 1000.0μg/ml respectively, process referring to the method in '4.2 Preparation of plasma samples'. Then inject 20μl of them into the chromatography system and record the chromatogram. The calibration curve is constructed by plotting the peak area ratios of theophylline to the internal standard versus the plasma concentration using least square regression.

4.5 Chromatographic conditions

Lichrospher ODS (250mm × 4.6mm × 5μm) or similar chromatographic column is used as the stationary phase. The mobile phase is a mixture of methanol and water (v/v = 50 : 50). The flow rate is 1.0ml/min and the column temperature is room temperature. The detection wavelength is 254nm and the injection volume is 20μl.

4.6 Determination of samples

Determine the samples under "Specificity" (blank plasma sample, theophylline – only plasma sample and internal standard – only plasma sample), respectively. There should be no endogenous interference of plasma on the internal standard and theophylline. The resolution between the internal standard and theophylline should meet the requirements and the number of theoretical plates is not less than 3000 according to the peak of theophylline.

Prepare plasma samples of series concentrations under "Calibration curve" and unknown test samples. Inject 20μl into the HPLC system and record the chromatogram. Substitute the peak area ratio of theophylline and the internal standard into the calibration curve and calculate the concentration of theophylline in the unknown sample according to the internal standard method.

5. Data recording and processing

5.1 Record for the sample preparation and experimental data

Table 14 – 1 Record for the sample preparation

Content	Specificity			Calibration curve					Unknown sample
Sample mark	0	0 + IS	0 + THP	1	2	3	4	5	X
Blank plasma	√	√	√	√	√	√	√	√	Test plasma
Theophylline	×	×	√	√	√	√	√	√	Blank methanol
Internal standard	×	√	×	√	√	√	√	√	√

√: Add   ×: Not added

Table 14 - 2　Record for theexperimental data

NO.	Simulation $C_{(THP)}$	THP		CAF		A_{THP}/A_{CAF}
		t_R	Peak area (A)	t_R	Peak area (A)	
Blank						
Blank + Internal Standard						
Blank + Theophylline						
1						
2						
3						
4						
5						
Unknown sample						

5. 2 The chromatograms of specificity.

5. 3 The evaluation of the calibration curve

Table 14 - 3　The evaluation of the calibration curve

	Simulation $C_{(THP)}$	A_{THP}/A_{CAF}	Calculated $C_{(THP)}$	Accuracy(%)
1				
2				
3				
4				
5				
Regression equation				

5. 4 Calculate the concentration of the unknown sample in plasma by regression equation

6. Discussion and guidance

6. 1 The purpose of specificity experiments

Specificity is also known as specialization, which means the ability of a method to detect the analyte in the presence of other "unrelated compounds" (non - specific interference) in the sample matrix. In this experiment, it is important to define the chromatographic peaks of theophylline and internal standard; and to judge whether endogenous substances in blank plasma interfere with chromatographic peaks of theophylline and the internal standard.

6. 2 The concept of "simulated drug blood concentration" in biopharmaceutical analysis

Pay attention that the response value should regress with "simulated drug blood concentration" instead of the concentration in the treated solution during injection or the concentration of the standard solution.

When prepare the calibration curve, a certain volume of the standard solution is added to a prescribed volume of blank plasma. When preparing unknown samples, in order to eliminate the error caused by the volume, blank methanol of the same volume should be supplemented.

6. 3 At the last step of the sample preparation

The supernatant was diluted with equal amount of mobile phase to avoid the "solvent effect", so as to obtain the satisfied peak shape.

6. 4 The use of pipette

a. When adjusting the range, if it is adjusted from a small volume to a large volume, you can first rotate the knob to the scale out of range, then back to the set volume to ensure the highest accuracy. Never screw the button out of the maximum range, otherwise it will jam the internal mechanical device and damage the pipette.

b. When assembling the tips, insert the pipette vertically. Make a slight rotation from left to right to tightly combine.

c. When pipetting the liquid, keep the pipette in a vertical state. Insert the tip $2 \sim 3$mm into the liquid surface. Pipetting the liquid several times to wet the tips in advance (especially when pipetting viscous liquids or liquids with different densities from water). Two methods of pipetting can be used: one is the forward pipetting method. Press the button to the first stop point with the thumb, then slowly release the button to suck the liquid back to the origin, and then press the button to the first stop to discharge the liquid, pause for a while and continue to press the button to the second stop to blow out the remaining liquid, and finally release the button. The second is reverse pipetting method. This method is generally used for transferring highly viscous liquids, biologically active liquids, easily foaming liquids or minimal amounts of liquids. The principle is to inhale more liquid than the set range, and is not necessary to blow out the residual when transferring. Press the button to the second stop and slowly release the button to the origin, then to the first stop point to discharge the liquid with the set range, keep the button at the first stop (never press down again), remove the tips and discard.

d. After use, hang it vertically on the pipette holder. When there is residual liquid in tips, do not put the pipette horizontally or inverted to avoid the liquid backflow and corrode the piston spring.

实验十五　液－液提取法考察血浆中茶碱的提取回收率

【实验目的】

1. 学习液－液提取法处理血浆的方法。
2. 学习提取回收率的考察方法。
3. 学习液－液提取法的应用范围。

【实验原理】

1. 液－液提取法简介　液－液提取法是常用的血浆样品前处理方法。多数药物是亲脂性的，在有机溶剂中的溶解度大于在水相中的溶解度，而血样中的内源性杂质多为强极性的水溶性物质，因而用有机溶剂提取即可除去大部分内源性杂质。应用液－液提取法时要考虑所选有机溶剂的极性，根据相似相溶原理选择，实际萃取时通常会加入第二种溶剂调整极性，提高选择性。溶剂的沸点应比较低、易挥散，毒性小。此外，应考虑溶剂与水的互溶性，常用溶剂乙醚中含 1.2% 水，可先用无水硫酸钠脱水。有机溶剂萃取次数通常为 1 次，必要时 2～3 次；有机溶剂用量与水体积比通常为 1∶1 或 2∶1，最佳提取次数与每次的溶剂用量要通过提取回收率确定。

液－液提取的浓集方法主要有两种，一种方法是在提取时加入的提取液尽量少，使被测组分提取到小体积溶剂中，然后直接吸出适量供测定。另一种方法是挥去提取溶剂法，挥去溶剂时应避免直接加热，防止被测组分破坏或挥发损失。挥去提取溶剂的常用方法是直接通入氮气流吹干；对于易随气流挥发或遇热不稳定的药物，可采用减压法挥去溶剂。

2. 提取回收率　提取回收率反映了样品处理过程中的提取效率，以样品提取和处理过程前后分析物含量百分比表示。样品处理方法的评价重点在于结果的精密度与重现性，而非待测物提取的完全与否。测定时需要制备高中低 3 个浓度的 QC 样品，制备至少 5 个独立的样品，另取空白生物介质，照 QC 样品同法处理，加入等量的标准溶液（必要时除去溶剂），同法处理高中低 3 个浓度的标准对照样品（含空白生物介质）。提取回收率又称绝对回收率，一般≥70% 就认为具有较好的提取回收率，80%～90% 则被大多数人认为是一个可接受的限度；如果某种药物提取回收率经试验各种溶剂后确实很难提高，低于 50% 也可接受，但重现性和精密度必须符合相关要求。低浓度的 RSD 应≤20%，中、高浓度 RSD 应≤15%。

【仪器与试剂】

1. 仪器　高效液相色谱仪，紫外检测器，氮气存储罐，微量注射器（10μl），分析天平，高速离心机，超声波清洗器，氮吹仪、恒温水浴锅、微量移液器（1000μl、200μl），涡旋混合振荡器，量瓶（100ml、10ml），量筒（500ml），离心管（5ml、1.5ml），吸液头（1000μl、100μl），移液管（5ml、1ml）。

2. 试剂　茶碱对照品（中国食品药品检定研究院），咖啡因对照品（中国食品药品检定研究院）；空白血浆、含药待测血浆；乙腈、乙酸乙酯为分析纯试剂，甲醇为色谱纯试剂，水为去离子水。

【实验内容】

1. 对照品溶液的制备

（1）茶碱对照品溶液　精密称取茶碱对照品100mg，置100ml量瓶中，用水溶解，并稀释制成每1ml含1000μg的对照品储备液，精密量取茶碱对照品储备液适量，用水稀释制成浓度分别为50.0、125.0、250.0、500.0和1000.0μg/ml的茶碱标准系列溶液，4℃冷藏。

（2）咖啡因内标溶液　精密称取咖啡因对照品10mg，置100ml量瓶中，用甲醇溶解，并定量稀释制成每1ml含100μg的储备溶液；精密量取该溶液1.0ml置100ml量瓶中，用甲醇稀释至刻度配成1μg/ml的标准溶液，4℃冷藏。

2. 样品处理方法

（1）提取回收率样品　取冷冻的血浆样品，在37℃水浴下解冻；精密吸取250μl，置2ml EP离心管中，精密加入内标溶液25μl，精密加入50.0、250.0和1000.0μg/ml的低、中、高3个浓度水平的茶碱对照品溶液各25μl，每个浓度水平5份，涡旋10秒混匀，加入乙酸乙酯0.8ml，涡旋混合3分钟，12000 rpm离心5分钟，分取上层有机相0.5ml，置于另一干燥的10ml离心管中，于50℃水浴中氮气流吹干，残渣加100μl流动相，涡旋3分钟使溶解，转移至1.5ml离心管中，12000 rpm离心2分钟，取上清液20μl进样，记录色谱图。

（2）提取回收率对照　照"提取回收率样品"方法制备空白血浆样品至"于50℃水浴中氮气流吹干"，残渣分别精密加入50.0、250.0和1000.0μg/ml的低、中、高3个浓度水平的茶碱对照品溶液及内标溶液各25μl，每个浓度水平2份，于50℃水浴中氮气流吹干，残渣加100μl流动相，涡旋3分钟使溶解，转移至1.5ml离心管中，12000 rpm离心2分钟，取上清液20μl进样，记录色谱图。

3. 色谱条件设置　色谱柱：Lichrospher ODS（250mm×4.6mm×5μm）或同类色谱柱；流动相：甲醇：水（50：50）；流速1.0ml/min；检测波长254nm；温度：室温；进样量：20μl。

【数据记录与处理】

1. 实验数据记录表

表15-1　实验数据记录和处理表

序号	茶碱		内标	
	t_R	峰面积 A	t_R	峰面积 A
样品1				
样品2				
样品3				
样品4				
样品5				
对照1				
对照2				

2. 提取回收率的计算　提取回收率按下式计算：茶碱提取回收率 $= A_s / A_{sr} \times 100\%$，内标提取回收率 $= A_i / A_{ir} \times 100\%$，其中 A_s 为样品溶液中茶碱的峰面积，A_i 为样品溶液中

内标的峰面积，A_{sr}为对照溶液中茶碱的峰面积，A_{ir}为对照溶液中内标的峰面积。

表 15 – 2 提取回收率计算表

	茶碱	内标
样品 1		
样品 2		
样品 3		
样品 4		
样品 5		
平均值		
RSD		

【讨论与指导】

1. 提取回收率与基质效应 提取回收率的对照样品，不能直接采用相应浓度的标准溶液，必须采用含有空白生物基质的相应浓度的样品，这是由于空白生物基质可能会对分析仪器信号产生抑制或增强（液质联用中特别明显）；而提取回收率的目的在于考察提取溶剂的萃取效率，所以需要消除空白生物基质对仪器响应的影响。生物基质中内源性物质对检测信号的影响，由"基质效应"这一验证项目进行考察。基质效应和提取回收率这两项验证项目有一定联系，但有本质区别，应注意区分。

2. 液 – 液提取法的注意事项

（1）溶剂蒸发所用的试管，底部应为尖锥形，这样可使最后数微升溶剂集中在管尖，既起到富集作用，又便于吸取。

（2）在萃取溶剂挥干并用流动相复溶时，常会出现混浊（脂肪类物质）。此时，应离心后取上清液进样，以保护色谱柱。

（3）液液提取法处理生物样品时易产生乳化问题，解决措施：轻缓振摇；萃取剂水中加入少量 NaCl；轻微乳化时，离心使分开；乳化严重时，置低温冰箱使水相快速冻凝，破坏乳化层，再融化后离心。

Experiment 15 Study on the Recovery of Theophylline in Plasma by Liquid – liquid Extraction

1. Experimental Purposes

1. 1 To learn the liquid – liquid extraction method for the plasma treatment.

1. 2 To learn the determination method of extraction recovery.

1. 3 To learn the application range of the liquid – liquid extraction method.

2. Experimental principles

2. 1 Introduction of Liquid – liquid extraction

Liquid – liquid extraction is a conventional separation and purification method. Many drugs are lipophilic and more soluble in organic solvents than in the aqueous phase. However, most of the endogenous interferences are water – soluble, so hydrophilic impurities can be removed by organic solvent extraction. The properties of organic solvent should be considered during the process of extraction according to the like dissolves like theory. In practice, a second solvent is usually added to adjust the polarity and improve the selectivity with a relatively low boiling point and toxicity and is easy to be volatilized and concentrated. In addition, the mutual solubility of solvent and water should be focused on. Ether is commonly used solvent in which usually contains 1. 2% water. It should be dehydrated with anhydrous sodium sulfate before use. Extracting with organic solvent usually perform once and 2 ~ 3 times if necessary. Volume ratio of organic solvents to water is usually 1 : 1 or 2 : 1. Optimum extraction times and the amount of solvent added per time are decided by the extraction recovery.

There are two major methods for the enrichment in liquid – liquid extraction. One method is to use as little volume of solvent as possible in the last extraction so that the analytes can be extracted into a relatively smaller volume, and then directly inject appropriate amount for assay. The other method is to volatilize the solvent. Direct heating should be avoided in case of destructing or volatilizing of the analytes. Blowing the solvent directly with a nitrogen stream is commonly adopted. Volatilization under reduced pressure is applied for components with volatility or thermal instability.

2. 2 Extraction recovery

Extraction recovery reflects the extraction efficiency in sample processing procedures, expressed as a percentage of the analyte content before and after the process of sample extraction and treatment. Evaluation of the sample processing method focuses more on the precision and reproducibility of the results than on the completeness of analyte extraction. At least 5 independent QC samples of 3 concentration levels (low, medium and high) should be prepared for determination. Meanwhile, the corresponding standard reference samples of 3 concentration levels (containing blank biological medium) are prepared by adding an equal amount of standard solution (removing the solvent if necessary) to blank biological medium with reference to QC samples.

Extraction recovery is also referred to as the absolute recovery. Generally, extraction recovery should exceed 70% and between 80% and 90% is an acceptable criterion. If the recovery of a drug is difficult to improve after extracted by various solvents, lower than 50% criterion is acceptable but the reproducibility and precision should meet the relevant requirements. *RSD* of extraction recovery at low concentration level should not exceed 20%, and that at the medium and high concentration level should not exceed 15%.

3. Apparatus and Reagents

3. 1 Apparatus

High performance liquid chromatography system with UV Detector; Microliter syringe (10μl); Storage tank for nitrogen; Analytical balance; Centrifuge; Ultrasonic cleaning instrument; Vortex mixer; Micropipettor(1000μl, 200μl); Volumetric flask (100ml, 10ml); Graduated cylinder (500ml); Centrifuge tubes(5ml, 1. 5ml); Pipet tips(1000μl, 100μl); Transfer pipette (5ml, 1ml).

3. 2 Reagents

Theophylline reference substance (National institute for the control of pharmaceutical and biological products); Caffeine reference substance (National institute for the control of pharmaceutical and biological products); Blank plasma; Acetonitrile and ethyl acetate is analytical reagent; Methanol is HPLC grade reagent; Water is deionized.

4. Experimental contents

4. 1 Preparation of the standard solution

Standard solution of theophylline: Accurately weigh 100mg of theophylline reference substance to a 100ml volumetric flask, dissolve and diluent with water to volume to prepare a stock solution of theophylline (1000μg/ml). The stock solution is further diluted with water to obtain standard solutions of 50. 0,125. 0,250. 0,500. 0 and 1000. 0μg/ml respectively. The stock and standard solutions are all stored at 4℃ in the refrigerator.

Standard solution of caffeine: Accurately weigh 10mg of caffeine reference substance to 100ml volumetric flask, dissolve with methanol to make a stock solution of caffeine (100μg/ml). The stock solution is further diluted with methanol obtain standard solution of 1. 0μg/ml. Keep at 4℃ for further use.

4. 2 Preparation of test samples

Extraction recovery sample Thaw the frozen plasma samples in 37℃ water bath. Precisely pipette 250μl of it to a 2ml EP tube. Add 25μl of the internal standard solution and 25μl of theophylline standard solution at 50,250 and 1000μg/ml corresponding to low, medium and high concentration levels. 5 replicates are prepared per concentration level. Vortex for 10 s to mix well, add 0. 8ml of ethyl acetate, then vortex for 3min and centrifuge at 12000 rpm for 5min. Transfer 0. 5ml of the upper organic phase to another 10ml dry centrifuge tube. Dry up at 50℃ water bath with a nitrogen stream. The residues are reconstituted in 200μl of the mobile phase, then vortexed for 3min to dissolve, and transferred to a 1. 5ml centrifuge tube. Inject 20μl of the supernatant into the chromatography system and record the chromatogram after centrifuging at 12 000 rpm for 2min.

Reference sample of extraction recovery The blank plasma sample is prepared referring to "Extraction recovery sample" until the step of "Dry up at 50℃ water bath with a nitrogen stream". Add 25μl of the internal standard solution and 25μl of theophylline standard solution at 50,250 and 1000μg/ml corresponding to low, medium and high concentration levels to the residue. 2 replicates are prepared per concentration level. Dry up at 50℃ water bath with a nitrogen stream. The residues are added with 100μl mobile phase, vortexed for 3min to dissolve, and transferred to a 1. 5ml centrifuge tube. Centrifuge at 12000 rpm for 2min. Inject 20μl of supernatant and record the chromatogram.

4. 3 Chromatographic conditions

Lichrospher ODS (250mm × 4. 6mm × 5μm) or similar chromatographic column is used as the stationary phase. The mobile phase is a mixture of methanol and water (v/v = 50∶50). The flow rate is 1.0ml/min and the column temperature is room temperature. The detection wavelength is 254nm and the injection volume is 20μl.

5. Data recording and processing

5.1 The record of experimental data

Table 15 – 1   The record of experimental data

NO.	THP		CAF	
	t_R	Peak Area (A)	t_R	Peak Area (A)
Sample 1				
Sample 2				
Sample 3				
Sample 4				
Sample 5				
Reference 1				
Reference 2				

5.2 Extraction recovery is calculated by the following formula：

$$\text{Extraction recovery of sample} = A_s / A_{sr} \times 100 \%$$

$$\text{Extraction recovery of the internal standard} = A_i / A_{ir} \times 100\%$$

Where, A_s is the peak area of theophylline in the sample solution; A_i is the peak area of the internal standard in sample solution; A_{sr} is the peak area of theophylline in standard solution; A_{ir} is the peak area of the internal standard in standard solution.

Table 15 – 2   Extraction recovery

	THP	CAF
Sample 1		
Sample 2		
Sample 3		
Sample 4		
Sample 5		
Average of recovery		
RSD of recovery		

6. Discussion and guidance

6.1 The difference between extraction recovery and matrix effect

Adopt samples of corresponding concentration containing the blank biological matrix as extraction recovery reference sample instead of standard solution of corresponding concentration due to the inhibited or enhanced signal of the analytical instrument by the blank biological matrix (especially in liquid chromatography – mass spectrometry). Extraction recovery aims to investigate the extraction efficiency of the solvent. Therefore, this experiment requires to eliminate the influence of the blank biological matrix on the instrument response. To evaluate the influence of endogenous substances on the detection signal in the biological matrix, verification project "Matrix Effect" is carried out. Matrix effect and the extraction recovery have certain relations but are essentially different. Attention should be paid to distinguish.

6.2 Notes for extraction recovery

a. Tubes with a conical bottom should be used for volatilization in order to concentrate and collect the sample.

b. The turbidity (fatty matter) is often generated after volatilization the extraction solvent and reconstitution in the mobile phase. The solution should be centrifuged and the supernatant is injected into HPLC in order to protect the column.

c. The phenomenon of emulsification is easy to generate while biological samples are treated with liquid – liquid extraction. Solutions include: shaking gently; adding a little NaCl into the extractant water; centrifugating to separate in case of mild emulsification occurs; freezing water phase quickly to destroy the emulsified layer if the emulsification is severe and then centrifugate after thawing.

实验十六 固相萃取法测定血浆中兰索拉唑的浓度

【实验目的】

1. 学习固相萃取法处理血浆样品的方法。

2. 学习体内药物分析中标准曲线的加权回归方法。

3. 学习测定血浆中兰索拉唑浓度的方法和步骤。

【实验原理】

1. 兰索拉唑简介 兰索拉唑（图 16 – 1）是一类抗酸性药物，是辅助用于消化性溃疡、反流性食管炎等疾病的药物；化学名为 2 – [[[3 – 甲基 – 4 – (2, 2, 2 – 三氟乙氧基) – 2 – 吡啶基] 甲基] 亚磺酰基] – 1H – 苯并咪唑，按干燥品计算，含 $C_{16}H_{14}F_3N_8O_2S$ 不得少于 99.0%。类白色至淡黄褐色的结晶性粉末；无臭，遇光及空气易变质。在二氯甲烷、甲醇、乙醇或丙酮中略溶，在醋酸乙酯中微溶，在水中不溶。兰索拉唑遇光不稳定，实验过程中应避免强光直射。

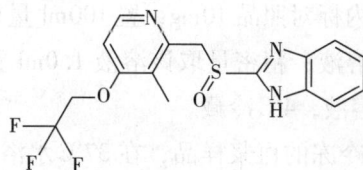

图 16 – 1 兰索拉唑（Lansoprazole）

2. 固相萃取的原理 将不同填料作为固定相装入微型小柱，当含有药物的生物样品溶液

扫码"学一学"

扫码"看一看"

通过时，由于受到吸附、分配、离子交换或其他亲和力作用，药物或杂质被保留在固定相上，用适当溶剂清洗杂质后，再用适当溶剂洗脱药物。最常用的 C_{18} 填料的固相萃取实验步骤如下：第一步：用 6~10 倍体积甲醇润湿小柱，活化填料；第二步：用 6~10 倍体积水或适当的缓冲液冲洗小柱，除去残留的甲醇；第三步：加样，使样品经过小柱，弃取废液；第四步：用水或适当的缓冲液冲洗小柱，去除内源性杂质，通空气或 N_2 干燥固相；第五步：选择适当的洗脱溶剂洗脱分析物，收集洗脱液，挥干溶剂，备用或直接进行在线分析。

固相萃取方法处理生物样品，最大的优势在于可以实现自动化操作，此外所需样品量少，可以避免液－液提取法中乳化现象；但缺点也同样明显，成本高昂，样品处理步骤繁琐，批与批之间有差异。

3. 加权最小二乘法回归标准曲线　用普通最小二乘法求算回归直线时，是以在标准曲线范围内每个浓度的测量方差来自同一总体为前提，所以对标准曲线上的每个浓度点的绝对误差赋予同等的重要性（权重系数 $W = 1$）。但在体内药物分析中，标准曲线浓度范围跨度大，其测量值的方差通常来自不同总体，所以会导致低浓度区域的浓度计算误差偏大，难以满足规定要求（$RE \leqslant \pm 15\%$，$RSD \leqslant 15\%$）。为了克服这一局限性，可在回归时引入一个权重因子（$W = 1/c$ 或者 $1/c^2$），增加低浓度点对标准曲线的贡献量，修正了回归方程，提高了低浓度点计算时的准确度。

加权最小二乘法的计算可以在 Excel 中自行编制相关公式计算，也可使用专业软件计算。注意观察采用权重系数后的回归结果和普通回归结果的差异。

【仪器与试剂】

1. 仪器　高效液相色谱仪，紫外检测器，氮气存储罐，微量注射器（10μl），分析天平，高速离心机，超声波清洗器，氮吹仪、恒温水浴锅、微量移液器（1000μl、200μl），涡旋混合振荡器，量瓶（100ml、10ml），量筒（500ml），离心管（5ml、1.5ml），吸液头（1000μl、100μl），移液管（5ml、1ml），固相萃取小柱。

2. 试剂　兰索拉唑对照品（中国食品药品检定研究院），吲达帕胺（中国食品药品检定研究院）；空白血浆、含药待测血浆；甲醇为色谱纯试剂，水为去离子水。

【实验内容】

1. 对照品溶液的制备

（1）兰索拉唑对照品溶液　精密称取兰索拉唑对照品 40mg，置 100ml 量瓶中，加甲醇溶解，并稀释制成每 1ml 含 400μg 的对照品储备液，精密量取兰索拉唑对照品储备液适量，用甲醇稀释制成浓度分别为 100.0、200.0、400.0、800.0、2000.0 和 4000.0ng/ml 的兰索拉唑标准系列溶液，4℃冷藏。

（2）内标溶液　精密称取内标对照品 10mg，置 100ml 量瓶中，用甲醇溶解，并定量稀释制成每 1ml 含 100μg 的储备溶液；精密量取该溶液 1.0ml 置 100ml 量瓶中，用甲醇稀释至刻度配成 1000ng/ml 的标准溶液，4℃冷藏。

2. 血浆样品处理方法　取冷冻的血浆样品，在 37℃ 水浴下解冻，精密吸取 200μl，置 1.5ml EP 管中，精密加入内标溶液 25μl，精密加入空白甲醇溶液 25μl（如果 QC 样品，替换为 25μl 相应浓度的系列对照品溶液），涡旋 10 秒混匀待用。

另取固相萃取小柱，用 4ml 甲醇活化，再用 4ml 纯化水清洗，上血浆样品过柱，用 4ml

纯化水清洗血浆内源性杂质，通空气干燥小柱，再用 2ml 甲醇洗脱待测物，收集甲醇洗脱液于 10ml 干燥离心管中，于 50℃水浴中氮气流吹干，残渣加 100μl 流动相，涡旋 3 分钟使溶解，转移至 1.5ml 离心管中，12000 rpm 离心 2 分钟，取上清液 20μl 进样，记录色谱图。

3. 标准曲线的制备 取空白血浆 200μl，分别置 2ml EP 管中，精密加入 100.0、200.0、400.0、800.0、2000.0 和 4000.0ng/ml 的拉索拉唑标准系列溶液各 25μl，按"血浆样品处理"项下同法处理，进样 20μl，记录色谱。以兰索拉唑血浆浓度为横坐标，兰索拉唑与内标的峰面积比值为纵坐标，用 $1/C^2$ 权重最小二乘法进行回归运算，求得的直线回归方程即为标准曲线。

4. 未知样品的浓度测定 取待测血浆样品，按"血浆样品处理"项下同法处理，进样 20μl，记录色谱图。将拉索拉唑与内标的峰面积比值代入标准曲线，按内标法求算未知样品的兰索拉唑的血药浓度。

5. 色谱条件设置 色谱柱：Lichrospher ODS（250mm × 4.6mm × 5μm）或同类色谱柱；流动相：甲醇：水（65：35）；流速 1.0ml/min；检测波长 285nm；温度：室温；进样量：20μl。

【数据记录与处理】

1. 实验数据记录表

表 16-1 实验数据记录表

序号	模拟 $C_{(LSP)}$	LSP		IS		A_{LSP}/A_{IS}
		t_R	峰面积 A	t_R	峰面积 A	
空白						
1						
2						
3						
4						
5						
6						
未知样品						

2. 使用加权最小二乘法对标准曲线进行回归，得到回归方程，并计算相关系数和标准曲线中每一个浓度点的准确度，判断准确度是否符合相关要求。

表 16-2 标准曲线回归方程的评价

	模拟 $C_{(THP)}$	A_{LSP}/A_{IS}	计算 $C_{(THP)}$	准确度（%）
1				
2				
3				
4				
5				
6				
回归方程				

3. 利用标准曲线回归方程计算未知样本中的药物浓度

【讨论与指导】

1. 最低定量限　最低定量限反映了方法的灵敏度，在保证具有一定可靠性（准确度与精密度符合要求）的前提下，该方法能够准确测定生物样品中药物的最低浓度，一般去以/N = 10 时的样品浓度作为的 LLOQ 估计值。在体内药物分析中，LLOQ 一般为标准曲线上的最低浓度点。

2. 交叉污染　在处理生物样品时应注意避免高浓度样品对低浓度样品的交叉污染，方法有：①样品处理时由低浓度到高浓度；②常用的对照品溶液、内标溶液、沉淀剂、提取溶剂、复溶流动相等液体试剂避免直接从大瓶取用，可分小包装使用；③移液器的枪头应垂直悬空于 EP 离心管上方，避免触碰 EP 离心管内壁；④对照品加样时用的微量注射器最好每个浓度点分别配备，否则，应保证交叉吸取不同浓度溶液时清洗干净；⑤自动进样器进样时是否在进样针上存在残留污染也是需要考察的关键点；⑥氮气吹干时应注意控制气流大小，太大会导致液体溅出，太小又影响干燥速度，应注意避免把氮气出口深入液面以下造成污染。

Experiment 16　Determination of Lansoprazole in Plasma by Solid Phase Extraction Method

1. Experimental Purposes

1.1 To learn the method for treating plasma sample by solid phase extraction.

1.2 To learn the weighted regression method for calibration curve in biopharmaceutical analysis.

1.3 To learn the experiment on the determination of lansoprazole in plasma.

2. Experimental principles

2.1 Introduction of lansoprazole

Lansoprazole（Fig. 16 – 1）is an antacid that is assisted in the treatment of peptic ulcer, reflux esophagitis or other diseases. Lansoprazole is 2 – [[[3 – methyl – 4 – (2,2,2 – trifluoroethoxy) – 2 – pyridyl]methyl]sulfinyl] – 1H – benzimidazole. It contains not less than 99.0% of lansoprazole（$C_{16}H_{14}F_3N_3O_2S$）, calculated on the anhydrous basis. As white to brownish white crystalline powder, lansoprazole is odorless and easily deteriorates when exposed to light and air. It is sparingly soluble in chloroform, methanol, ethanol or acetone, slightly soluble in ethyl acetate, practically insoluble in water. Lansoprazole is unstable under light, avoiding direct sunlight during the processes.

2.2 The principle of the solid phase extraction

Load different stuffs as stationary phase into the micro – column. When the biological sample solution containing drug passes through the micro – column, the drug or impurities are retained on

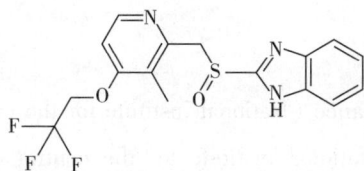

Fig. 16 – 1 Lansoprazole, LSP

the stationary phase based on adsorption, distribution, ion exchange or other affinity. Removing the impurities with an appropriate solvent, then the drug can be desorbed by another appropriate solvent. The following are the solid phase extraction experimental procedures with ODS C18column. The first step: wetting the micro – column with 6 – 10 volumes of methanol to activate the sorbent; the second step: washing the micro – column with 6 – 10 volumes of water or appropriate buffer solution to remove the residual methanol; the third step: loading the sample onto the micro – column and discarding the waste; the fourth step: washing the micro – column with water or buffer solution to remove endogenous impurities and drying the column with air or N_2; The fifth step: eluting the analytes with an appropriate solvent, collecting the eluate and evaporating the solvent for later or online analysis.

The advantages of solid phase extraction in the treatment of biological samples are easy automation, less sample usage, and no emulsification. However, this method is costly, the sample treatment is cumbersome, and the column has inter – batch variation.

2. 3 Regress the calibration curve by weighted least square method

The precondition of establishing a regression line by least squares is that the variance of each concentration within the range of the calibration curve comes from one population. The absolute error of each point on the calibration curve is equally important (W = 1). However, due to the large concentration range of the calibration curve, the data usually comes from different populations in the biopharmaceutical analysis. Therefore, the error in the low concentration region is too large to meet the requirements (RE $\leqslant$ ± 15% , RSD $\leqslant$ 15%). In order to overcome this limitation, a weighting factor (W = 1/c or $1/c^2$) can be introduced to increase the contribution of the low concentration point to the calibration curve. This method corrects the regression equation and improves the accuracy of low concentrations.

The calculation of the weighted least square method can be carried out by establishing formula in Excel, or using professional software. Observe the difference of the results between using the weight coefficient and the ordinary least squares method.

3. Apparatus and Reagents

3. 1 Apparatus

High performance liquid chromatography system with UV Detector; Microliter syringe (10μl) ; Storage tank for nitrogen; Analytical balance; Centrifuge; Ultrasonic cleaning instrument; Vortex mixer; Micropipettor(1000μl, 200μl) ; Volumetric flask (100ml, 10ml) ; Graduated cylinder (500ml) ; Centrifuge tubes (5ml, 1. 5ml) ; Pipet tips (1000μl, 100μl) ; Transfer pipette (5ml, 1ml) ; Solid phase extraction column.

3. 2 Reagents

Lansoprazole reference substance (National institute for the control of pharmaceutical and biological products) ; Indapamide (National institute for the control of pharmaceutical and biological products) ; Blank plasma ; Methanol is HPLC grade reagent ; Water is deionized.

4. Experimental content

4. 1 Preparation of the standard solution

Lansoprazole standard solutionWeigh about 40mg of lansoprazole reference substance, accurately, to a 100ml volumetric flask, dissolve and dilute with methanol to volume and mix to prepare 400μg/ml stock solution of lansoprazole. The stock solution is further diluted with methanol to obtain standard solutions of 100. 0, 200. 0, 400. 0, 800. 0, 2000. 0 and 4000. 0ng/ml. Keep at 4℃ for further use.

Internal standard solution Weigh about 10mg of the internal standard reference, accurately, to a 100ml volumetric flask, dissolve and dilute with methanol to volume and mix to prepare 100μg/ml stock solution. Accurately pipette 1ml of this solution to a 100ml volumetric flask. Dilute it with methanol to volume and mix it to prepare 1000ng/ml standard solution. Keep at 4℃ for further use.

4. 2 The processing method of plasma sample

Thaw the frozen plasma sample under 37℃ water bath. Transfer accurately 200μl of it to a 1. 5ml EP tube, precisely add 25μl of internal standard solution and 25μl of methanol solution (if it is QC sample, replace it with 25μl of corresponding concentration of standard solution) , vortex for 10s.

Activate the solid phase extraction column with 4ml of methanol and 4ml of purified water. Plasma samples are passed through the column and endogenous impurities are removed by 4ml of purified water. Dry the column with air and elute the analyte with methanol. Then collect the eluent in a 10ml dry centrifuge tube and evaporate it to dryness in 50℃ water bath under a gentle stream of nitrogen. The residues are reconstituted in 100μl of the mobile phase. Vortex the mixture for 3min and transfer it to a 1. 5ml centrifuge tube and centrifuge at 12000 rpm for 2min. Then 20μl of the supernatant is injected and the chromatogram is recorded.

4. 3 Preparation of calibration curve

To each of 200μl of blank plasma in 2ml EP tubes, add 25μl of a series of lanso – prazole standard solution 100. 0, 200. 0, 400. 0, 800. 0, 2000. 0 and 4000. 0ng/ml, respecttively. Process them in the same way as directed under the "The processing method of plasma sample". Then 20μl of the sample is injected and the chromatogram is recorded. The calibration curve is constructed by plotting the peak area ratios of each analyte to the internal standard versus the concentration using weighed least square method.

4. 4 Determination of the sample solution

Process the plasma sample in the same way as directed under the "The processing method of plasma sample". And then $20\mu l$ of sample is injected and the chromatogram is recorded. Substituting the peak area ratio of lansoprazole to the internal standard into the calibration curve. The concentration of lansoprazole in the plasma sample is calculated by the internal standard method.

4. 5 Chromatographic conditions

Lichrospher ODS ($250mm \times 4.6mm \times 5\mu m$) or similar chromatographic column is used as the stationary phase. The mobile phase is a mixture of methanol and water ($v/v = 65 : 35$). The flow rate is 1.0ml/min and the column temperature is room temperature. The detection wavelength is 285nm and the injection volume is $20\mu l$.

5. Data record and processing

5. 1 The record of experimental data

Table 16 – 1 The record of experimental data

NO.	$C_{(LSP)}$	LSP		IS		A_{LSP}/A_{IS}
		t_R	Area	t_R	Area	
Blank						
1						
2						
3						
4						
5						
6						
Sample						

5. 2 Calculate the regression equation and correlation coefficient of the calibration curve by weighted least squares method. Verify whether the accuracy of each point meets the requirements.

Table 16 – 2 The evaluation of the calibration curve

	Simulation $C_{(LSP)}$	A_{LSP}/A_{IS}	Calculated $C_{(LSP)}$	Accuracy(%)
1				
2				
3				
4				
5				
6				
Regression equation				

5. 3 Calculate the plasma concentration of the sample by the regression equation

6. Discussion and guidance

6. 1 Lower Limit of Quantification

Lower Limit of Quantification (LLOQ) reflects the sensitivity of the method. It represents the lowest amount of an analyte in a sample that can be quantitatively determined with predefined precision and accuracy. The concentration at S/N = 10 is generally regarded as the estimation of LLOQ. In biopharmaceutical analysis, LLOQ is the lowest concentration on the calibration curve.

6. 2 Crossover

It is critical to avoid the crossover between high and low concentration samples when treating biological samples. The methods include: (a) Treat samples from low concentration to high concentration; (b) Liquid reagents such as reference solution, internal standard solution, precipitant, extraction solvent, and mobile phase should be taken in small packages; (c) The pipette tip should be suspended vertically above the EP centrifuge tube to avoid touching the inner wall of the EP centrifuge tube; (d) Use different microliter syringe for each concentration point when adding standard solutions, otherwise, the microliter syringe should be cleaned; (e) Pay attention to the residual on the syringe when the autosampler injects continuously; (f) Control the flow rate of nitrogen. Too much nitrogen will make the liquid splashed out, too little will slow down the drying speed. In addition, the nitrogen outlet should not be reached into the liquid, avoiding cross contamination.

扫码"练一练"

第五章　色谱联用技术在药物分析中的应用

Chapter 5　Application of hyphenated chromatographic techniques in pharmaceutical Analysis

实验十七　气质联用法鉴定维生素 E 软胶囊

【实验目的】

1. 学习气质联用仪的基本操作步骤。

2. 学习气质联用法鉴定药物的原理。

3. 学习 EI 离子源的工作原理。

【实验原理】

1. 维生素 E 性状　维生素 E 是一系列苯并二氢吡喃衍生物的总称，天然维生素 E 有多种存在形式，根据甲基数目和位置及是否含有双键可将其分为 α -、β -、γ -、δ - 生育酚和生育三烯酚，其中 α - 生育酚生物效价最高。由于生育酚性质活泼不稳定，因此，在其各种制剂中一般采用更稳定的酯化形态，目前广泛使用于软胶囊中的是 α - 生育酚醋酸酯。

维生素 E 胶丸是一种富含天然型/人工型维生素 E（图 17 - 1）的软胶囊，具有自由基清除、抗氧化活性的作用，临床上使用主要是起协同作用，和其他药物联合使用。本品为微黄色至黄色或黄绿色澄清的黏稠液体；几乎无臭；遇光色渐变深。本品在无水乙醇、丙酮、乙醚或植物油中易溶，在水中不溶。

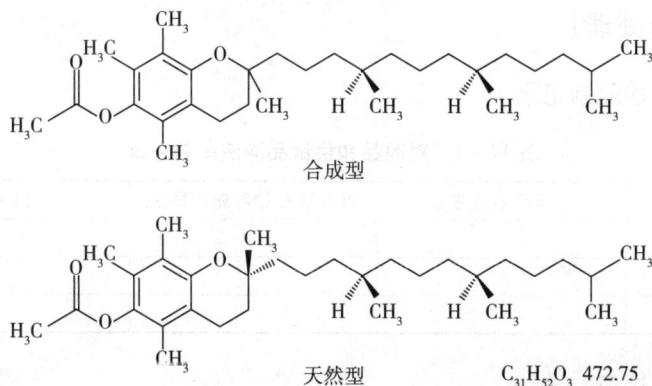

合成型

天然型　$C_{31}H_{52}O_3$　472.75

图 17 - 1　合成型和天然型维生素 E 的化学结构式

2. 气质联用的原理　气质联用（GC - MS）又叫气相色谱 - 质谱联用技术，它以气相色谱作为高效分离系统，质谱为检测系统。样品在质谱部分被离子化后，经质谱质量分析器将离子碎片按质量数分开，经检测器获得质谱图。气相色谱的优势在于分离高效，为混合物的

139

分离提供了最有效的选择，但难以获得物质的结构信息，定性时无法给出确定的结论。

传统质谱能够提供物质结构信息，样品用量少，分析样品通常需要进行纯化，达到一定的纯度要求，才可以直接进行分析。

气质联用技术体现了色谱和质谱优势的互补，色谱高分离能力结合质谱高选择性、高灵敏度分析能力，能够提供相对分子质量与结构信息。广泛应用于药物分析、食品分析和环境分析，生命分析等许多领域。

【仪器与试剂】

1. 仪器 气相色谱－质谱联用仪，高纯氦气，分析天平，棕色容量瓶（10ml），尼龙滤头，气相进样针（1μl）。

2. 试剂 维生素 E 对照品，维生素 E 软胶囊（市售），正己烷为分析纯试剂。

【实验内容】

1. 对照品溶液的配制 取维生素 E 对照品约 20mg，精密称定，置 10ml 棕色容量瓶中，加正己烷稀释至刻度，密塞摇匀，作为对照品溶液。

2. 供试品溶液的配制 取装量差异项下的内容物，混合均匀，取适量（约相当于维生素 E 20mg），精密称定，置 10ml 棕色容量瓶中，加正己烷稀释至刻度，密塞摇匀，作为供试品溶液。

3. 色谱－质谱条件的设置 气相色谱柱：以 HP－5 MS（30m×0.25mm×0.25μm）毛细管柱或同类型色谱柱；载气：氦气；柱内流量：2.0ml/min；分流比：1∶10；进样口温度：300℃；程序升温（起始温度 200℃，保持 2 分钟，以 20℃/min 速率升温至 300℃，保持 6 分钟）；进样 1μl。

质谱条件：接口温度 300℃；离子源温度 200℃；电子轰击能量 70eV；离子监测扫描范围（m/z 35~500）；采集延时 3 分钟。

4. 定性分析 取对照品和供试品溶液各 1μl 进行 GC－MS 分析，获得总离子流图，记录色谱峰的保留时间和相应的质谱总离子流图。

【数据记录与处理】

1. 对照品溶液的配制记录

表 17－1 对照品和供试品溶液配制记录

对照品称样量	对照品溶液浓度	维生素 E 软胶囊称样量	供试品溶液浓度

2. GC－MS 色谱图

表 17－2 保留时间数据记录

	t_R（维生素 E）（min）
对照品溶液	
供试品溶液	

3. 维生素 E 的质谱特征

表 17 – 3 维生素 E 的质谱特征峰

总离子流 t_R	m/z	m/z	m/z	m/z	m/z	m/z
维生素 E 对照品						
维生素 E 胶丸						

【讨论与指导】

1. 气质联用技术的优点 仅利用气相色谱的保留时间来对化合物进行定性鉴别的方法具有一定的局限性，存在假阳性的可能，证据不够充分。如果使用气质联用或者液质联用技术，通过与对照品比对色谱保留时间，母离子分子量和碎片离子分子量一致，可获得有力的证据来鉴定药物及其杂质。

2. 电子轰击离子化（EI）的原理 电子轰击离子化（EI）是最常用的一种离子源，有机分子被一束电子流（能量一般为 70eV）轰击，失去一个外层电子，形成带正电荷的分子离子（M^+），M^+ 继续受到电子轰击而引起化学键的断裂或分子重排，进一步碎裂成各种碎片离子、中性离子或游离基，在电场作用下，正离子被加速、聚焦、进入质量分析器分析。故 EI 电离是一种单分子的裂解反应，属于硬电离方法。

3. 硬电离质谱与软电离质谱的区别 一般认为 LC – MS 多采用的是软电离方式。虽然硬电离质谱中讨论的裂解反应理论亦基本适用于软电离质谱的裂解反应。但软电离质谱电离条件与硬电离质谱不同，因而生成的产物离子不同。诸如硬电离质谱生成奇电子的分子离子 M + ·，而软电离质谱生成偶电子的准分子离子，通常为［M + H］$^+$ 或［M – H］$^-$ 等，二者母离子的质量和带电荷状态不同。EI 裂解反应大都在离子源内的电离过程中发生，并以自由基诱发开裂（α 裂解）为主。软电离条件下，母离子在离子源内基本不发生裂解反应（APCI 除外），大都通过多级质谱技术采用碰撞诱导引起解离（CID），并以正电荷诱发开裂（i 裂解）为主。此外，在 CID 作用下的多级质谱中，由于母离子仅为单一同位素的离子，因此，不存在同位素离子峰，从而与硬电离单级全扫描质谱特征不同。故同一化合物的硬电离质谱和软电离质谱是绝然不同的。

4. 软电离质谱中的裂解 ESI 和 APCI 属于软电离方法，主要形成准分子离子，因此易于得到样品分子量。为得到进一步的结构信息，可使待测离子与惰性气体原子（如氩气）进行碰撞诱导解离（collision – induced dissociation，CID），又称为碰撞活化断裂（collision – activated dissociation，CAD）或简称碰撞活化（collisional activation，CA）。通过调节惰性原子的能量，可以使被碰撞的离子产生不同程度裂解的质谱。在空间串联的多级质谱（三重四极质谱等）中，一般可测得二级质谱（母离子→子离子），此碰撞诱导解离需要在独立的碰撞池（collision cell）内进行，三重四极质谱中的第二重四极主要发挥碰撞池功能。

Experiment 17   Identification of Vitamin E Soft Capsules by Gas Chromatography – Mass Spectrometry

1. Experimental Purposes

1. 1 To learn the operation of gas chromatography – mass spectrometry (GC – MS).

1. 2 To learn the principles of GC – MS for the identification of drugs.

1. 3 To learn the working principle of the EI ion source.

2. Experimental principle

2. 1 The Characters of Vitamin E

Vitamin E is a general term for a series of benzodihydropyran derivatives. Natural vitamin E has various forms. It can be divided into α – 、β – 、γ – 、δ – and tocotrienol according to the number and position of methyl groups and whether it contains double bonds, wherein α – tocopherol has the highest bioavailability. Since the tocopherol is active and unstable, a more stable esterification form is generally employed in various preparations, and α – tocopheryl acetate is currently widely used in soft capsules.

Vitamin E capsule is a kind of soft capsule rich in natural/synthetic vitamin E (Fig. 17 – 1). It has the function of free radical scavenging and anti – oxidation activity. And it is mainly used in clinical practice and in combination with other drugs. This product is a viscous liquid with a yellowish to yellow or yellowish green clarification; almost odorless; the color gradually darkens after illumination. This product is easily soluble in anhydrous ethanol, acetone, ether or vegetable oil and is insoluble in water.

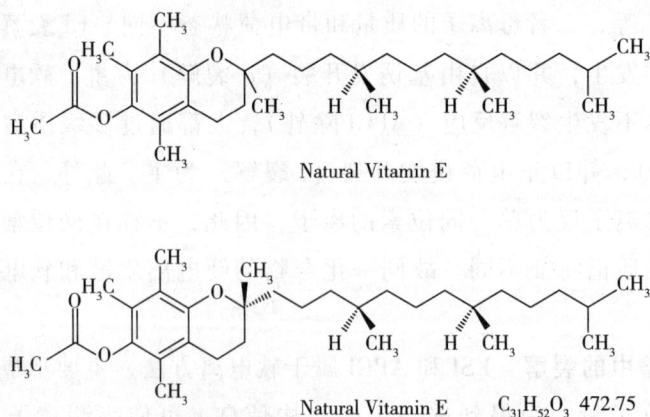

Natural Vitamin E

Natural Vitamin E $C_{31}H_{52}O_3$ 472.75

Fig. 17 – 1   The molecular structure of synthetic and natural vitamin E

2. 2 Principle of GC – MS

GC – MS uses gas chromatography as a high – efficiency separation system and mass spectrometry as a detection system. After the sample is ionized in the mass spectrometer, mass analyzer separates the ion fragments, and a mass spectrum is obtained through the detector.

The advantage of gas chromatographyis the efficient separation, which provides the most effective choice for the separation of mixtures. However, it is difficult to obtain structural information of the substances, and it is impossible to draw a definite conclusion in qualitative analysis. Traditional mass spectrometry can provide structural information of a substance and the amount of sample used is small, but the target sample to be analyzed needs to be purified to meet a certain purity requirement and then the analysis can be directly performed.

GC – MS technology embodies the complementary advantages of chromatography and mass spectrometry, combining the high separation ability of chromatography with complex samples with MS's high selectivity, high sensitivity and the ability to provide relative molecular mass and structural information. And GC – MS has been widely used in many fields such as pharmaceutical analysis, food analysis and environmental analysis, life analysis and many other fields.

3. Apparatus and Reagents

3. 1 Apparatus

Gas chromatography – mass spectrometer; High purity helium; Analytical balance; Brown volumetric flask (10ml); Nylon filter head; Gas phase syringe (1μl).

3. 2 Reagents

Vitamin E reference (China National Institute for the Control of Pharmaceutical and Biological Products); Vitamin E soft capsule (commercially available); n – hexane is analytical reagent (AR).

4. Experimental contents

4. 1 Preparation of thereference solution

Accurately weigh 20mg of vitamin E reference substance to a 10ml brown volumetric flask, dilute it with n – hexane to the mark and shake well before use.

4. 2 Preparation of the sample solution

The contents are mixed evenly, then accurately weigh the appropriate amount (about 20mg of vitamin E) to a 10ml brown volumetric flask, dilute it with n – hexane to the mark and shake well before use.

4. 3 Setting of GC – MS conditions

GC conditions: HP – 5MS (30m × 0. 25mm × 0. 25μm) or similar chromatographic column is used as the stationary phase. The carrier gas is helium. The column flow is about 2ml/min and the split ratio is 1 : 20. The temperature of the inlet is 300℃. The column temperature is set according to the program: the initial temperature is 200℃, hold for 2min; then the temperature is increased to 300℃ at the rate of 20℃/min, hold for 6min. The inject volume is 1μl.

MS conditions: interface temperature is 300℃. The ion source temperature is 200℃. The electron bombardment energy is 70 eV. The ion monitoring scanning range is m/z 35 ~ 500. The acquisition delay is 3min.

4. 4 Qualitative Analysis

Take 1μl of reference solution and the sample solution for GC – MS analysis respectively to obtain the total ion chromatogram and record the retention time of vitamin E.

5. Data record and processing

5. 1 Record for the preparation of the sample solution

Table 17 – 1   Record for the preparation of the sample solution

The amount of reference substance	The concentration of the reference solution	The amount of the Vitamin E soft capsule	The concentration of the sample solution

5. 2 GC – MS chromatogram

Table 17 – 2   Record for retention time

Sample	t_R (Vitamin E) (min)
The reference solution	
The sample solution	

5. 3 Mass spectral of vitamin E

Table 17 – 3   Mass spectral of vitamin E

	Total ion current(t_R)	m/z	m/z	m/z	m/z	m/z	m/z
Vitamin E reference							
Vitamin E capsule							

6. Discussion and guidance

6. 1 Advantages of GC – MS technology

Qualitative analysis by the retention time is not enough for the identification of drug and its impurities. The false positives are often found due to the insufficient evidence only by the retention time. For GC – MS or LC – MS method, besides the retention time, the parent ion molecular weight and the fragment ion molecular weight also can be used for the identification. Therefore, GC – MS and LC – MS can provide strong evidence to identify the type of drug and their impurities.

6. 2 Principle of electron bombardment ionization (EI)

Electron bombardment ionization (EI) is one of the most commonly used ion sources. Organic molecules are bombarded by a stream of electrons (generally 70eV), losing an outer electron, forming a positively charged molecular ion (M^+), M^+ continue to be bombarded by electrons to cause chemical bond rupture or molecular rearrangement, further fragmentation into various fragment ions, neutral ions or radicals. Under the action of electric field, positive ions are accelerated, focused, and analyzed by mass analyzer. Therefore, EI ionization is a single – molecule cleavage reaction and belongs to the hard ionization method.

6.3 The difference between the hard ionization and the soft ionization

Generally, the ionization in LC – MS is the soft ionization mode. Although the theory of cleavage reactions in hard ionization is applicable for the cleavage reaction of soft ionization, the soft ionization conditions are different from the hard ionization conditions. For example, hard ionization mass spectrometry generates molecular electrons M + · of odd electrons, while soft ionization mass spectrometry generates adduct ions of even electrons, usually $[M + H]^+$ or $[M - H]^-$, etc. Therefore, their mass spectra are quite different. Most of EI cracking reactions occur in the ionization process of ion source, and mainly in the free radical induced cracking (alpha cracking). In the soft ionization, the parent ions basically do not undergo cracking reaction in the ion source (except APCI). Most of them adopt collision induced dissociation (CID) by inert atoms in multistage mass spectrometry, and mainly crack induced by positive charge (i cracking). In addition, in the multistage mass spectrum under the action of CID, since the parent ion is only the ion of a single isotope, there is no isotope ion peak, which is different from in the hard ionization with the single – stage full – scan mass spectrum. Therefore, the hard ionization mass spectra and soft ionization mass spectra of the same compound are absolutely different.

6.4 Dissociation in the soft ionization mass spectrometry

ESI and APCI are soft ionization methods that mainly form parent ions, so it is easy to obtain the molecular weight of the sample. In order to obtainthe further structural information, the parent ions can be collided – induced dissociation (CID) by the atoms of inert gases such as argon, which also known as collision – activated dissociation (CAD) or collision activation (CA). By modulating the energy of inert atoms, the collided ions can be subjected to mass spectrometry with varying degrees of cleavage. In a spatially connected multi – stage mass spectrometer (triple quadrupole mass spectrometer,), a two – stage mass spectrum (parent ion → daughter ion) can generally be measured, and this collision – induced dissociation needs to be performed in a separate collision cell. The second quadrupole in the quadrupole mass spectrum primarily functions as a collision cell.

实验十八　高效液相色谱 – 质谱法测定人血浆中甲磺酸伊马替尼的验证

【实验目的】

1. 学习高效液相色谱 – 质谱联用法（液质联用）的使用。
2. 学习液质联用法测定血浆样本的验证方法。
3. 学习亲水作用色谱的分离原理。

扫码"学一学"

【实验原理】

1. 甲磺酸伊马替尼的性状　甲磺酸伊马替尼（Imatinib mesylate）是由瑞士诺华公司研制的一种酪氨酸激酶抑制剂，商品名格列卫（Gleevec），用于治疗慢性骨髓性白血病、胃肠道基质肿瘤等癌症的第一代靶向药物。甲磺酸伊马替尼的结构式如图 18 – 1 所示，其纯品为白色粉末，分子量为 589.71，熔点 226℃，极易溶于水。由于甲磺酸伊马替尼化学结

构中含有吡啶环、哌啶环和氮原子等极性较大的碱性基团，酸性流动相中其在常规的反相键合相色谱柱上保留较弱，不利于建立血浆中含量测定的高灵敏度方法，因此本实验采用了亲水作用色谱进行分离测定。

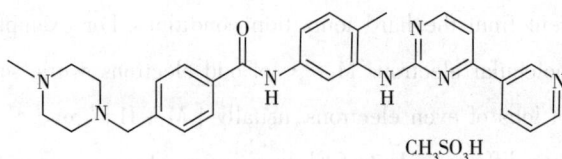

图 18 – 1　甲磺酸伊马替尼的结构

2. 液质联用仪的构造　液质联用仪主要由液相色谱系统、样品导入系统、接口（interface）、质量分析器、离子检测器、真空系统和计算机数据处理系统等组成（图 18 – 2）。样品通过 LC 色谱分离后，首先在接口中离子化（离子化是指样品以液相离子的形式转变成气相离子的过程），生成的气相离子通过质量分析器按 m/z 的大小顺序得以分离，并通过离子检测器将离子信号转化为电信号，再经电子倍增器放大，检测信号放大后传输至计算机数据处理系统。真空系统能够保证质谱仪在高真空状态下工作，减少本底的干扰，避免发生不必要的分子 – 离子反应。计算机控制仪器的所有功能，并完成数据处理。

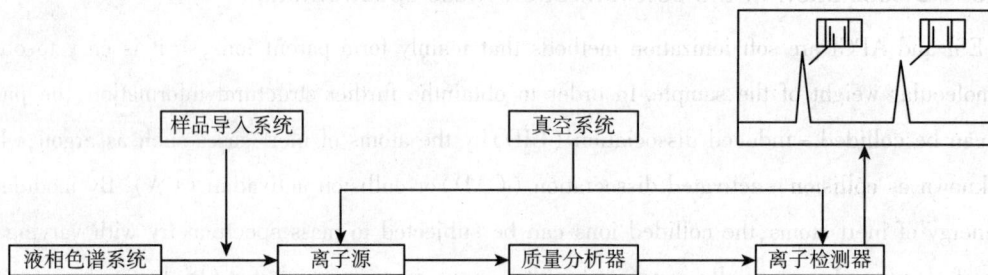

图 18 – 2　液质联用仪的组成图

【仪器与试剂】

1. 仪器　高效液相色谱仪（配有自动进样器），三重四极杆质谱，分析天平，微量注射器（100μl），量瓶（10ml），移液管（1ml）。

2. 试剂　甲磺酸伊马替尼对照品（纯度：≥99%），伊马替尼 – d8 对照品（内标，纯度：≥99%），甲磺酸伊马替尼片（规格：100mg/片），水为超纯水，甲醇、乙腈、甲酸、甲基叔丁基醚等均为色谱纯。

【实验内容】

1. 对照品溶液的配制　取甲磺酸伊马替尼对照品约 10mg，精密称定，置 10ml 量瓶中，加甲醇/水（1∶1）溶液溶解并稀释至刻度，摇匀，作为储备液。精密量取甲磺酸伊马替尼储备液适量，用甲醇/水（1∶1）溶液逐级稀释制成 50.0、100、500、2500、5000、10000、15000 和 20000ng/ml 的甲磺酸伊马替尼系列工作液，备用。

取伊马替尼 – d8 对照品约 10mg，精密称定，置 10ml 量瓶中，加甲醇/水（1∶1）溶液溶解并稀释至刻度，摇匀，作为储备液。精密量取内标储备液适量，用甲醇/水（1∶1）混合溶液逐级稀释制成 50ng/ml 的内标工作液，备用。

2. 人血浆样品处理　取冷冻的血浆样品，于37℃水浴下解冻，精密吸取50μl，置2ml具塞离心管中，加入内标溶液20μl，加入650μl甲基叔丁基醚，涡旋混匀，于4℃条件下10000rpm离心5分钟，取上清液200μl至96孔板中，35℃氮气流下吹干；加入300μl流动相复溶，涡旋离心后，取5.0μl上清液进样分析。

3. 色谱质谱条件的设置　色谱柱：$ZIC^{©}$ – HILIC（150mm × 4.6mm × 5μm）或同类型色谱柱；流动相：水（含0.4%甲酸，pH为3.2）– 乙腈；梯度洗脱（表18 –1）；流速：0.4ml/min；柱温：40℃，进样量：5.0μl。

表18 –1　流动相的梯度洗脱条件

时间（min）	0	0.7	1.9	2.0	2.1	3.1	3.2	4.1	4.2	5.5
乙腈（%）	70	70	70	70	50	50	95	95	70	Stop
切换阀（位置）		MS	Waste							

质谱条件：伊马替尼分子结构中含有碱性氮原子，在电喷雾离子化（正离子模式）方式下有很好的质谱响应，采用多反应监测（MRM）扫描方式。甲磺酸伊马替尼和内标伊马替尼 – d8 的监测离子对分别为 m/z 494.3→217.3 和 m/z 502.3→225.2；碰撞能量、喷雾电压、电离温度等参数由仪器自动方式优化获得。

4. 方法学验证

（1）专属性　取6批不同来源的空白血浆和空白血浆加标样品，按"人血浆样品处理"项下处理后，分别进样10μl，记录甲磺酸伊马替尼及内标的保留时间，观察空白血浆基质对于待测物和内标的干扰。

（2）标准曲线　取50μl空白血浆样品8份，置于2ml离心管中，分别精密加入系列浓度的甲磺酸伊马替尼工作液5μl，涡旋10秒，混匀。按"人血浆样品处理"项自"加入内标溶液20μl"起，同法处理，进样10μl，记录色谱图。以甲磺酸伊马替尼血浆浓度为横坐标，甲磺酸伊马替尼与内标的峰面积比值为纵坐标，用加权最小二乘法进行回归运算，求得回归方程即为标准曲线。

（3）精密度与准确度　取空白血浆样品50μl，按"标准曲线"项下方法制成最低定量限、低、中、高（5.0、10.0、500、2000ng/ml）4个浓度的质控（QC）样品，每一浓度平行5个样品分析；根据标准曲线计算QC样品中甲磺酸伊马替尼的实测浓度，以此计算本法的精密度与准确度。

（4）提取回收率　取空白血浆样品50μl，按"标准曲线"项下方法制成低、中、高（10.0、500、2000ng/ml）3个浓度的QC样品，每一浓度水平5个样品。同时，取空白血浆样品50μl，按"人血浆样品处理"项下的方法操作，获得空白血浆的提取液吹干后的流动相复溶液，配制成低、中、高3个浓度的对照溶液。计算两组待测物溶液中各浓度水平待测物的峰面积比值计算提取回收率。

（5）基质效应　取6批不同来源的空白血浆，对每批基质，用空白血浆的提取液吹干后的流动相复溶液配制成低、高（10.0、2000ng/ml）2个浓度的样品。同时，取低、高2个浓度水平等量的甲磺酸伊马替尼对照品溶液。计算两组待测物溶液中各浓度水平待测物的峰面积比值计算基质效应。

（6）稳定性试验　按标准曲线测定方法配制低、高（10.0、2000ng/ml）2个浓度的QC样品血浆样品，模拟实际血浆样品在存储、运输、操作、进样过程中的可能环境。考察样品稳定性。

【数据记录与处理】

1. 溶液的配制记录

表 18-2　对照品溶液的配制记录

名称	称样量（W）	储备液浓度（Cs）
甲磺酸伊马替尼对照品		
伊马替尼 - d8 对照品		

2. 专属性测定结果

（1）空白血浆色谱图

（2）空白血浆加标样品色谱图

3. 标准曲线测定结果

表 18-3　标准曲线的测定结果

序号	甲磺酸伊马替尼		内标		浓度
	保留时间（min）	峰面积	保留时间（min）	峰面积	
1					
2					
3					
4					
5					
6					
7					
8					

4. 精密度与准确度测定结果

表 18-4　精密度与准确度的结果

序号	QC 浓度							
	最低定量限		低		中		高	
	实测值（ng/ml）	准确度（%）	实测值（ng/ml）	准确度（%）	实测值（ng/ml）	准确度（%）	实测值（ng/ml）	准确度（%）
1								
2								
3								
4								
5								
平均值								
RSD（%）								

5. 提取回收率与基质效应测定结果

表 18 − 5　提取回收率的测定结果

	序号	QC 浓度					
		低		中		高	
		实测值 (ng/ml)	回收率 (%)	实测值 (ng/ml)	回收率 (%)	实测值 (ng/ml)	回收率 (%)
回收率样品	1						
	2						
	3						
	4						
	5						
回收率对照	1						
	2						
平均值							
RSD (%)							

表 18 − 6　甲磺酸伊马替尼基质效应的测定结果

序号	QC 浓度			
	低		高	
	基质样品 (峰面积)	基质对照 (峰面积)	基质样品 (峰面积)	基质对照 (峰面积)
1				
2				
3				
4				
5				
6				
平均值				
RSD (%)				
基质效应				

6. 稳定性测试结果

表 18 − 7　稳定性测试的结果

	序号	QC 浓度			
		低		高	
		实测值 (ng/ml)	准确度 (%)	实测值 (ng/ml)	准确度 (%)
立即测定	1				
	2				
	3				

续表

	序号	QC 浓度			
		低		高	
		实测值 （ng/ml）	准确度 （%）	实测值 （ng/ml）	准确度 （%）
室温放置 6h 后测定	1				
	2				
	3				
进样器放置 24h 后测定	1				
	2				
	3				
3 次冻融 循环后测定	1				
	2				
	3				

【讨论与指导】

1. HILIC 的特点 亲水作用色谱（HILIC）提供了一种与传统反相色谱（RPLC）互补的保留方式，能够为在 RPLC 上保留较弱或没有保留的物质提供合适的保留；药物在 HILIC 柱上的洗脱顺序与 RPLC 柱的正好相反，极性较大的物质后出峰，极性较小的物质先出峰。目前，HILIC 的固定相材料日益丰富，涵盖了未衍生化硅胶、氨基、氰基、二醇基、酰胺型、聚琥珀酰亚胺型、糖型和两性离子型键合相等；其典型的流动相是由水或挥发性缓冲盐溶液与 40% ~97% 的乙腈组成。因此，HILIC 柱对极性药物保留较强，且流动相中较高的有机相比例能显著提高质谱响应。

2. 液质联用的接口 液质联用的关键是接口技术。大气压电离接口（API）是目前应用最广泛的接口技术，包括电喷雾离子化（ESI）和大气压化学离子化（APCI）。APCI 采用电晕放电方式使流动相离子化，形成单电荷准分子离子，适用于中低极性且有一定挥发性的小分子化合物。ESI 利用离子蒸发实现液相离子化，易形成多电荷离子，适用于极性化合物和生物大分子，适用范围要大于 APCI。

API 为软电离技术，一般得到准分子离子信息，缺乏碎片离子的结构信息；可以通过串联质谱（MS/MS）技术而获得更多结构信息。LC - MS/MS 在定性定量方面都显示出无比的优越性，其特点为高分辨、低噪音、高通量，可以研究结构和碎片反应，并可直接分析多组分混合物。

3. 基质效应 基质效应（Matrix effect）是指在样品检测过程中，有待测物以外的其他物质的存在，直接或间接影响待测物响应的现象。由于质谱检测的高选择性，基质效应的影响在色谱图上往往观察不到，即空白基质色谱图表现为一条直线，但这些共流出组分会改变待测物的离子化效率，引起对待测物检测信号的抑制或提高。这些基质成分包含了生物样品中的内源性成分和样品前处理过程中引入的外源性成分。

4. 内标的选择 内标定量法可以有效减小样品前处理以及分析过程中引入的误差，从而保证分析结果的准确性。通常，以质谱为检测器进行定量分析时，待测物的稳定同位素标记物是首选的内标物质；若商品化的同位素内标不易获得（如价格昂贵），亦可选择待测物的结构类似物作为内标物质，但此时，需要从保留时间、质谱响应、基质效应等方面对候选物质进行考察。

Experiment 18　Validation for the Determination of Imatinib Mesylate in Human Plasma by High Performance Liquid Chromatography – Mass Spectrometry

1. Experimental purposes

1.1 To learn the operation of high performance liquid chromatography – mass spectrometry (LC – MS).

1.2 To learn the validation for the analysis of plasma samples by LC – MS.

1.3 To learn the separation principle of hydrophilic interaction chromatography.

2. Experimental principles

2.1 The characters of imatinib mesylate

Imatinib mesylate (Fig. 18 – 1) is a tyrosine kinase inhibitor developed by Novartis AG of Switzerland with the trade name Gleevec. It is a first – generation targeted drug for the treatment of cancers such as chronic myelogenous leukemia and gastrointestinal stromal tumors. Its pure product is white powder with molecular weight of 589.71 and melting point of 226℃. It is very soluble in water. Since the chemical structure of imatinib mesylate contains the relatively polar basic groups such as pyridine ring, piperidine ring and nitrogen atoms, it is weakly retained on the conventional reversed – phase bonded phase chromatography columns, which is not conducive to the establishment of a highly sensitive method for determination of its plasma concentration. Therefore, this experiment uses hydrophilic interaction chromatography for separation and determination.

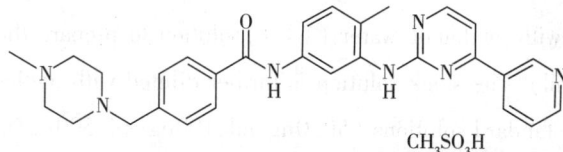

Fig. 18 – 1　Structure of imatinib mesylate

2.2 Construction of LC – MS

The LC – MS is mainly composed of a liquid chromatography system, an injection system, an interface, a mass analyzer, an ion detector, a vacuum system, and a data processing system (Fig. 18 – 2). After the separation by liquid chromatography, the sample is first ionized in the interface, and the generated gas phase ions are separated by mass analyzer in the order of m/z. Then the ion signal is converted into an electrical signal by an ion detector, amplified by an electron multiplier, and transmitted to a computer data processing system. The vacuum system ensures that the mass spectrometer operates under high vacuum conditions, reducing background interference and avoiding unwanted molecular – ion reactions. The computer controls all the functions of the instrument and performs data processing.

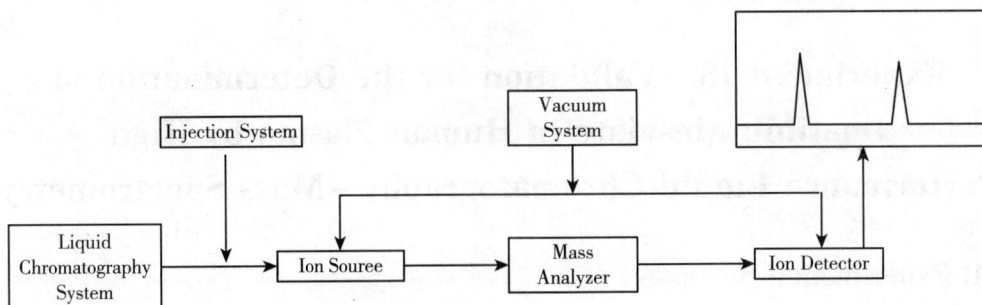

Fig. 18 – 2　Construction of LC – MS

3. Apparatus and Reagents

3. 1 Apparatus

High performance liquid chromatograph system (with autosampler); Triple quadrupole mass spectrometry; Analytical balance; Microsyringe (100μl); Volumetric flask (10ml); Transfer pipettes (1ml).

3. 2 Reagents

Imatinib mesylate reference substance (purity is more than 99%); Imatinib mesylate – d8 reference substance (purity is more than 99%); Imatinib mesylate tablets (Specification: 100mg/tablet); Methanol and acetonitrile are HPLC grade reagent; Formic acid and methyl tert – butyl ether are analytical reagent (AR); Water is deionized.

4. Experimental contents

4. 1 Preparation of the reference solution

Accurately weigh 10mg of imatinib mesylate reference substance to a 10ml volumetric flask, then dissolve and dilute with methanol/water (1 : 1) solution to prepare the stock solution of imatinib mesylate (1. 0mg/ml). The stock solution is further diluted with methanol/water (1 : 1) solution to obtain a series of standard solutions (50. 0ng/ml, 100ng/ml, 500ng/ml, 2500ng/ml, 5000ng/ml, 10000ng/ml, 15000ng/ml and 20000ng/ml).

Accurately weigh 10mg of imatinib mesylate – d8 reference substance to a 10ml volumetric flask, then dissolve and dilute with methanol/water (1 : 1) solution to preparethe stock solution of imatinib mesylate – d8 (1. 0mg/ml). The stock solution is further diluted with methanol/water (1 : 1) solution to obtain the internal standard solution (50ng/ml).

4. 2 Preparation of the plasma sample

Thaw the frozen plasma samples at 37℃ water bath. Accuratelytransfer 50μl of it to a 2ml centrifuge tube, add 20μl of internal standard (imatinib mesylate – d8) solution and 650μl of methyl tert – butyl ether. Vortex the mixture for 5min and centrifuge at 10,000 rpm for 5min at 4℃. Take 200μl of the supernatant into a 96 – well plate and blow dry at 35℃ under nitrogen flow. Add

$300\mu l$ of mobile phase to reconstitute, vortex and centrifuge, and inject $5.0\mu l$ of the supernatant to the LC – MS system.

4.3 LC – MS conditions

LC conditions: Merck ZIC$^{©}$ – HILIC (150mm × 4.6mm × 5μm) or similar columns is used as the stationary phase. Water (containing 0.4% formic acid, pH 3.2) – acetonitrile are used as the mobile phase with the flow rate of 0.4ml/min and column temperature of 40℃. The elution gradient is shown in Table 18 – 1 and the injection volume is set to $5.0\mu l$.

Table 18 – 1　Gradient conditions of the mobile phase

Time (min)	0	0.7	1.9	2.0	2.1	3.1	3.2	4.1	4.2	5.5
Acetonitrile(%)	70	70	70	70	50	50	95	95	70	Stop
Switching Valve		MS	Waste							

MS conditions: Imatinib contains a basic nitrogen atom and has a good mass spectrometric response in electrospray ionization (positive ion mode) mode with multiple reaction monitoring (MRM). The MRM conditions of imatinib mesylate and internal standard are set to m/z 494.3→217.3 and m/z 502.3→225.2, respectively. Other operating parameters, such as collision energy, spray voltage, and ionization temperature, are automatically optimized by the instrument.

4.4 Method Validation

a. Specificity　Take 6 batches of blank plasma and blank plasma spiked with reference substances from different sources, and process them in the same way as directed under the "Preparation of the plasma sample". After analysis, the peaks and peak areas of each chromatogram at the retention time of imatinib mesylate and the internal standard are recorded.

b. Calibration curve　To each of $50\mu l$ of blank plasma in 2ml centrifuge tubes, add $5\mu l$ of a series of imatinib mesylate standard solution 50.0ng/ml, 100ng/ml, 500ng/ml, 2500ng/ml, 5000ng/ml, 10000ng/ml, 15000ng/ml and 20000ng/ml, respectively. Then process them in the same way as directed under the "Preparation of the plasma sample" beginning with "add $20\mu l$ of internal standard". After analysis, the chromatograms are recorded. The calibration curve is constructed by plotting the peak area versus the concentration using weighted linear least square regression.

c. Precision and Accuracy　To each of the 2ml centrifuge tubes, add accurately $50\mu l$ of blank plasma. The quality control (QC) samples are prepared according to the "Calibration curve" at concentrations of the lowest limit of quantitative, low, medium and high (5.0, 10.0, 500 and 2000ng/ml) with 5 replicates at each concentration. The concentration of imatinib mesylate in QC samples are calculated according to the calibration curve. The precision and accuracy are determined with the measured concentration of the QC samples.

d. Recovery　QC samples at low, medium and high (10.0, 500, and 2000ng/ml) concentration levels of 5 replicates are prepared according to the "Calibration curve". Meanwhile, the corresponding samples are prepared by adding the imatinib mesylate standard solutions and internal standard post extraction (n = 2). The recovery is determined by comparing the peak areas of the analytes in plasma samples that have been spiked with the analytes prior to extraction with those of the samples to which the analytes have been added post – extraction.

e. Matrix effect　The imatinib mesylate standard solutions with low and high concentrations (10. 0 and 2000ng/ml) are prepared in mobile phase. Meanwhile,6 blank sample extracts from different sources are prepared and spiked with the analyte at the same concentration levels. The matrix effect is evaluated by comparing the peak area of the analyte dissolved in the supernatant of the processed blank plasma to that of the standard solution dissolved in mobile phase.

f. Stability　QC samples at low and high (10. 0 and 2000ng/ml) concentration levels are prepared according to the "Calibration curve" to simulate the environment that real plasma samples may face during storage,transportation,preparation,and injection.

5. Data record and processing

5. 1 Record for the solution preparation

Table 18 –2　Record for the solution preparation

Substance	Amount	Concentration
Imatinib mesylate		
Imatinib mesylate – d8		

5. 2 Results of specificity

a. The typical chromatogram of blank plasma.

b. The typical chromatogram of blank plasma spiked with imatinib mesylate and the internal standard.

5. 3 Results of calibration curve.

Table 18 –3　Results of calibration curve

No.	Imatinib mesylate		Internal standard		Concentration
	Retention time (min)	Peak Area	Retention time (min)	Peak Area	
1					
2					
3					
4					
5					
6					
7					
8					

5. 4 Results of precision and accuracy

Table 18 – 4　Results of precision and accuracy

No.	QCConcentration							
	LLOQ		Low		Medium		High	
	Measured (ng/ml)	Accuracy (%)	Measured (ng/ml)	Accuracy (%)	Measured (ng/ml)	Accuracy (%)	Measured (ng/ml)	Accuracy (%)
1								
2								
3								
4								
5								
Mean								
RSD(%)								

5. 5 Results of recovery and matrix effect

Table 18 – 5　Results of recovery

	No.	QC Concentration					
		Low		Medium		High	
		Measured (ng/ml)	Recovery (%)	Measured (ng/ml)	Recovery (%)	Measured (ng/ml)	Recovery (%)
Sample	1						
	2						
	3						
	4						
	5						
Contrast	1						
	2						
Mean							
RSD (%)							

Table 18 – 6　Results of matrix effect

No.	QC concentration			
	Low		High	
	Sample (Peak Area)	Contrast (Peak Area)	Sample (Peak Area)	Contrast (Peak Area)
1				
2				
3				
4				
5				
6				
Mean				
RSD(%)				
Matrix effect				

5. 6 Results of stability test

Table 18 - 7   Results of stability test

	No.	QC concentration			
		Low		High	
		Measured (ng/ml)	Accuracy (%)	Measured (ng/ml)	Accuracy (%)
Immediate determination	1				
	2				
	3				
Short - term (6h, room temperature)	1				
	2				
	3				
Post - preparative (24h,4℃)	1				
	2				
	3				
Freeze - thaw (three cycles, -20℃ - room temperature)	1				
	2				
	3				

6. Discussion and guidance

6. 1 Advantage of HILIC

Hydrophilic interaction chromatography (HILIC) provides a complementary method to tradition-al reversed - phase liquid chromatography (RPLC) which means it provides suitable retention for analytes that is weakly retained or unretained on RPLC. The elution order of the drug on the HILIC column is exactly the opposite of that of the RPLC column. The less polar substance is eluted first. At present, HILIC's stationary phase materials are increasingly abundant, including underiva tized silica gel, amino, diol, amide, polysuccinimide, and zwitterionic linkages. Its typical mobile phase consists of water or a volatile buffer solution with 40% ~97% acetonitrile. Therefore, the HIL-IC column has strong ability to retain polar drugs, and the high organic ratio in the mobile phase can significantly increase the mass spectral response of the analyte.

6. 2 LC - MS interface

The interface is the key technology for LC/MS. Atmospheric pressure ionization (API) is current-ly the most widely used interface technology. These ionization methods include electrospray ionization (ESI) and atmospheric pressure chemical ionization (APCI). APCI uses a corona discharge method to ionize the mobile phase to form a single - charged quasi - molecular ion, which is suitable for small - molecule compounds with low to medium polarity and certain volatility. ESI uses ion evaporation to a-chieve liquid phase ionization, which is easy to form multi - charged ions. It is suitable for polar com-pounds and biomacromolecules, and its application range is much larger than APCI.

The API is a soft ionization technique, which generally obtains excimer ion information and lacks structural information of fragment ions; more structural information can be obtained by tandem mass spectrometry (MS/MS). LC – MS/MS shows unparalleled superiority in both qualitative and quantitative analysis, characterized by high resolution, low noise, and high throughput. It can be used for structural and fragmentation studies and can directly analyze multi – component mixtures.

6.3 Matrix effect

Matrix effect refers to the phenomenon that the response of the analyte is directly or indirectly affected by the presence of other coeluting components during the sample detection process. Due to the high selectivity of mass spectrometry, the influence of matrix effect is often not observed on the chromatogram, that is, the blank matrix chromatogram shows a straight line. However, these co – eluting components may change the ionization efficiency of the analyte, causing its signal to be suppressed or increased. These matrix components consist of endogenous components in the biological sample and exogenous components introduced during sample preparation.

6.4 Selection of internal standard

The internal standard method can effectively reduce the error introduced in the sample pretreatment and analysis process, thus ensuring the accuracy of the analysis results. Generally, when quantitative analysis is performed by mass spectrometry as a detector, a stable isotope label of the analyte is the preferred internal standard substance. If the commercial isotope internal standard is not easy to obtain (such as too expensive), the structural analog of the analyte may be selected as the internal standard substance. But at this time, the candidates need to be examined from the aspects of retention time, mass spectrometry response, and matrix effect.

实验十九　高效液相色谱－质谱法测定川楝子中川楝素的含量

扫码"学一学"

【实验目的】

1. 学习高效液相色谱－质谱法条件的建立与优化过程。
2. 学习高效液相色谱－质谱法测定川楝子中川楝素含量的方法。
3. 学习药物含量测定方法学验证的项目和内容。

【实验原理】

1. 川楝素的性状　川楝子为楝科植物物川楝 *Melia toosendan* Sieb. et Zucc. 的干燥成熟果实，亦称"金铃子"，其作为传统中药在临床应用十分广泛。《本草纲目》记载该药性味苦寒，有小毒，有酸味，入肝、胃、小肠经。现代药理学研究表明，川楝子具有驱蛔杀虫、抗肿瘤、抗病毒、抗氧化、抑制破骨细胞、镇痛等作用。

川楝子中主要成分是三萜类、挥发油、黄酮类、脂肪酸、酚酸类和多糖等化合物。其中，楝科特征性成分楝烷型三萜由于其复杂多变的化学结构和昆虫拒食性等特点，引起了较多关注。川楝素（Toosendanin，图19－1）是一种代表性楝烷型三萜类化合物，其纯品为白色或类白色结晶性粉末，分子式为 $C_{30}H_{38}O_{11}$，分子量为574.62。其易溶于吡啶、丙酮、乙醇、甲醇，微溶于氯仿、苯，几乎不溶于石油醚和水。熔点为 178~180℃（稀乙醇）或

238～240℃（95%乙醇）。旋光度为－13.1°（c＝1.75，丙酮）。《中国药典》（2020年版）规定，川楝子中川楝素的含量为0.060%～0.20%。

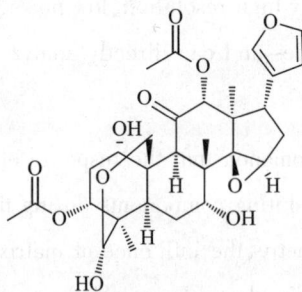

图19-1　川楝素（Toosendanin）的结构

2. 质谱定量分析　质谱（Mass spectrometry）是一种电离化学物质并根据其质荷比（m/z）对其进行排序的分析技术。质谱法测定药物含量时，可采用选择离子监测模式（Selected-ion monitoring，SIM）、选择反应监测模式（selective reaction monitoring，SRM）或多反应监测模式（multi reaction monitoring，MRM），以外标法或内标法定量。采用标准曲线法时，测定相同体积的系列标准溶液在m/z离子处的响应值，以响应值为纵坐标，标准溶液浓度为横坐标，绘制标准曲线，获得回归方程。按规定制备供试品溶液，测定其在特征m/z离子处的响应值，带入标准曲线或回归方程计算，得到待测物的浓度。

【仪器与试剂】

1. 仪器　高效液相色谱仪（配有自动进样器），三重四极杆质谱，分析天平，离心机，超声波清洗器，量瓶（50ml、10ml），圆底烧瓶（100ml），移液管（1ml）。

2. 试剂　川楝子（市售品）；川楝素对照品（中国药品生物制品检定所）；甲醇（色谱纯）、甲酸（色谱纯）、高纯氮气（纯度＞99.999%）、高纯氩气（纯度＞99.999%）、超纯水。

【实验内容】

1. 对照品溶液的制备　取川楝素对照品适量，精密称定，加甲醇制成每1ml约含川楝素100μg的对照品贮备液。精密量取1ml对照品贮备液，置50ml量瓶中，甲醇稀释至刻度，制成2μg/ml对照品溶液。

2. 供试品溶液的制备　取本品中粉（四号筛）约0.25g，精密称定，置100ml圆底烧瓶中，精密加入甲醇50ml，称定重量，加热回流1小时，放冷，再称定重量，用甲醇补足减失的重量，摇匀，微孔滤膜（0.22μm）滤过，取续滤液，即得。

3. 色谱条件　色谱柱：Hypersil GOLD C_{18}（50mm×2.1mm，3μm）或同类型色谱柱；流动相：乙腈-0.01%甲酸溶液（31∶69）；流速：0.2ml/min；柱温：35℃；进样量：2μl。

4. 质谱条件　电喷雾（ESI）离子源，负离子模式。脱溶剂气体为氮气，碰撞气体为氩气。碰撞能量、喷雾电压、电离温度等参数由仪器自动方式优化获得。根据川楝素对照品的保留时间与质谱征离子碎片信息进行定性和定量分析。

5. 条件选择和优化　取对照品溶液，按上述色谱与质谱条件进样，在m/z 100～800范围内，分别采用正、负离子模式进行全扫描，选择合适的电离模式与分子离子峰。以准分子离子峰为母离子，对其产生的碎片离子进行二级质谱扫描，选取丰度强且干扰较少的离子对作为定性和定量离子。参考监测离子对为m/z：573.3→425.3；m/z：573.3→531.4。

优化质谱参数，使质谱仪灵敏度达到最优。

6. 线性关系的考察　配置系列浓度为 0.05、0.25、0.50、1.00、5.00、10.00、50.00μg/ml 的标准工作溶液，按上述色谱与质谱条件进样测定。由于川楝素结构中存在半缩醛结构，始终存在 2 个互变异构体，因此以川楝素两个峰面积之和为纵坐标（Y），以对照品浓度为横坐标（X），绘制标准曲线，得线性回归方程。

7. 定量限和检测限　取川楝素对照品溶液用甲醇逐级稀释，按上述色谱与质谱条件进样测定，记录峰高（S）和基线噪音（N），以 S/N＝3 所对应的川楝素浓度确定检测限（LOD），以 S/N＝10 所对应的川楝素浓度确定定量限（LOQ）。

8. 精密度试验　取川楝子药材，按"2"项下制备 1 份供试品溶液，连续进样 6 次。记录川楝素的峰面积，计算 RSD 值，考察仪器精密度。

9. 重复性试验　取同一批次川楝子药材，按"2"项下平行制备 6 份供试品溶液，分别进样测定，计算 6 份供试品中川楝素的含量和 RSD 值，考察方法的重复性。

10. 稳定性试验　取川楝子药材，按"2"项下制备 1 份供试品溶液，分别于 0、1、2、4、8、12 和 24 小时，按上述色谱与质谱条件进样测定，记录川楝素的峰面积，计算 RSD 值，考察供试品溶液的稳定性。

11. 加样回收率试验　称取已知含量的川楝子药材共 9 份，每份约 0.12g，分别精密加入低、中、高不同含量的川楝素对照品（80μg、160μg 和 240μg），每个含量水平 3 份。按"2"项下制备供试品溶液，进样测定，计算回收率、平均回收率与 RSD 值。

12. 样品测定　取不同厂家的川楝子药材，精密称定，按"2"项下制备供试品溶液，进样测定，每个样品测定 3 次，以标准曲线法计算得到川楝素含量，考察不同厂家的川楝子药材是否符合药典规定要求。

【数据记录与处理】

1. 川楝子中川楝素的母离子与子离子选择

表 19－1　正、负离子模式的选择

模式	母离子（m/z）	子离子（m/z）
正离子模式		
负离子模式		

2. 线性范围、检出限和定量限

表 19－2　川楝素的线性关系考察

序号	浓度（μg/ml）	峰面积 A（mAU）
1		
2		
3		
4		
5		
6		
7		

标准曲线方程为：　　　　　　　　相关系数 r＝

检测限（LOD）：S/N＝3 对应的川楝素浓度为：

定量限（LOQ）：S/N＝10 对应的川楝素浓度为：

3. 精密度试验

表 19－3　精密度试验

序号	峰面积	平均峰面积	RSD（%）
1			
2			
3			
4			
5			
6			

4. 重复性试验

表 19－4　重复性试验

序号	取样量（g）	峰面积	川楝素含量（μg/g）	平均含量	RSD（%）
1					
2					
3					
4					
5					
6					

5. 稳定性试验

表 19－5　稳定性试验

放置时间（h）	峰面积	RSD（%）
0		
1		
2		
4		
8		
12		
24		

6. 加样回收率试验

表 19－6　加样回收率试验

序号	取样量（g）	样品含量（μg）	加入量（μg）	测得量（μg）	回收率（%）	平均回收率（%）	RSD（%）
1			80				
2			80				
3			80				
4			160				
5			160				
6			160				
7			240				
8			240				
9			240				

7. 样品测定

表 19 – 7　样品测定

序号	样品批号	取样量（g）	峰面积	含量（μg/g）
1				
2				
3				
4				
5				
6				

【讨论与指导】

1. 液质联用的流动相　流动相与样品需过微孔滤膜，流动相应超声脱气（或仪器装有在线脱气装置）以避免压力波动，流动相应及时更换。液质联用分析常用的流动相为甲醇、乙腈、水及缓冲盐溶液。液质联用操作中，应使用挥发性的缓冲盐如甲酸铵、乙酸铵，或挥发性酸碱如甲酸、乙酸或氨水。避免含磷和氯的缓冲液，含钠和钾的成分必须 <1mmol/L，因为盐含量过高会抑制离子源信号和堵塞喷雾针，污染仪器。禁止使用不挥发性酸碱如磷酸等。

2. 液质联用分析条件的选择和优化　液质联用分析时，应根据目标物的结构性质来选择正负离子化模式。正离子模式常适合于碱性样品，可用甲酸或乙酸对样品酸化，样品中含有仲氨或叔氨可优先考虑使用正离子模式（如磺胺类、喹诺酮类物质）。负离子模式适合于酸性样品，可用氨水对样品进行碱化，样品中含有较多的强负电性基团，如含氯、溴和多个羟基时可考虑负离子模式（如氯霉素）。

3. 常见的质谱扫描模式

（1）全扫描模式（Full Scan）　对指定质量范围内的离子扫描并记录其色谱图。质谱采集时，扫描设定的一段范围，例如 150 – 500amu。对于未知物的分析，首先采用该模式，初步获得该未知物的分子量。对于二级质谱（MS/MS）或多级质谱（MSn）检测时，首先采用全扫描模式以获得其碎片离子信息。

（2）产物离子扫描（Product – ion scan）　在第一级质量分析器中选择某 m/z 的离子作为前体离子，测定该离子在第二级质量分析器中、一定的质量范围内的所有碎片离子（产物离子）的质荷比与相对强度，获得该前体离子的质谱。

（3）前体离子扫描（Precursor – ion scan）　在第二级质量分析器中选择某 m/z 的产物离子，测定在第一级质量分析器中、一定的质量范围内所有能产生该碎片离子的前体离子。

（4）中性丢失扫描（neutral – loss scan）　以恒定的质量差异，在一定的质量范围内同时测定第一级、第二级质量分析器中的所有前体离子和产物离子，以发现能产生特定中性碎片（如 CO_2）丢失的化合物或同系物。

（5）选择离子监测模式（Selected – ion monitoring，SIM）　仅扫描设定的一个离子。常用于已知化合物的测定，可提高目标离子的灵敏度，并排除其他离子的干扰。

（6）选择反应监测模式（Selective reaction monitoring，SRM）　选择第一级质量分析器中的前体离子（m/z），测定该离子在第二级质量分析器中的特定产物离子（m/z）的强度，以定量分析复杂混合物中的低浓度待测化合物，可排除噪音等干扰，提高灵敏度和信噪比。

（7）多反应监测模式（Multi reaction monitoring，MRM） 同时检测两对及以上的前体离子－产物离子。在一级扫描下选择各个化合物特定的母离子，再将其碰撞碎裂后在二级扫描中分析其特定的碎片离子。

在建立含量测定方法时，顺序通常是：①采用全扫描模式获得化合物的分子量；②采用 SIM 模式，优化质谱电压等参数条件，保证母离子的传输效率；③采用子离子扫描，使用已优化电压，选择定量离子，并优化碰撞能量，优化子离子的响应；④采用 MRM 定量，优化每个子离子的碰撞能量。

4. 方法学验证 为证明采用的方法适合于相应检测要求，分析方法需经验证。需验证的分析项目有：鉴别试验、限量或定量检查、原料药或制剂中有效成分含量测定，以及制剂中其他成分（如防腐剂等，中药中其他残留物、添加剂等）的测定。验证指标有：准确度、精密度（包括重复性、中间精密度和重现性）、专属性、检测限、定量限。线性、范围和耐用性。在分析方法验证中，须采用标准物质进行试验。

Experiment 19　Determination of Toosendanin in Toosendan Fructus by High Performance Liquid Chromatography – Mass Spectrometry

1. Experimental purposes

1.1 To learn the condition establishment and method validation ofhigh performance liquid chromatography – mass spectrometry (LC – MS).

1.2 To learn the procedures for the assay of toosendanin by LC – MS.

1.3 To learn the items and parameters of analytical method validation.

2. Experimental principles

2.1 The characters of toosendanin

Toosendan Fructus, also known as "Jinlingzi", is the dry and ripe fruit of *Melia toosendan* Sieb. et Zucc. (Meliaceae). Nowadays it has been widely used in clinical application as a traditional Chinese medicine. The Compendium of Materia Medica records that the property and flavor are predominantly bitter – cold, slightly toxic, and enter to liver, intestine and bladder channels. Modern pharmacological studies have demonstrated that it possesses a variety of functions such as the roundworm elimination, antitumor, antivirus, anti – oxidation and analgesic effects.

Toosendan Fructus contains triterpenoids, volatile oils, flavonoids, aromatic fatty acids, phenolic acids, polysaccharides, and other chemical compositions. The most characteristic constituents in Meliaceae family are meliacane triterpenoids, which attract wide attention because of the complicated structures and antifeeding activities. The representative compound is toosendanin (Fig. 19 – 1), which is the white or almost white powder, with molecular formula of $C_{30}H_{38}O_{11}$ and molecular weight of 574.62. It is freely soluble in pyridine, acetone, ethanol and methanol, slightly soluble in chloroform and benzene, and practically insoluble in petroleum ether and water. the melting point is about 178 ~ 180℃ (dilute ethanol) or 238 ~ 240℃ (95% ethanol). Optical rotation is − 13.1° (c = 1.75, acetone). Toosendan Fructus contains 0.060% ~ 0.20% of toosendanin (Chinese Pharmacopoeia 2020, Volume Ⅰ).

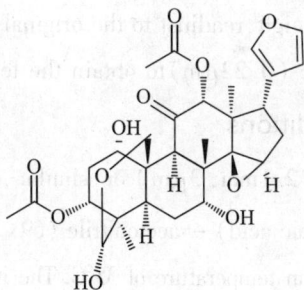

Fig. 19 − 1　Structure of toosendanin

2.2 Quantitative analysis by mass spectrometry

Mass spectrometry is based on the direct measurement of the ratio of the mass to the number of positive or negative elementary charges of ions (m/z) obtained from the substance to be analysed. In pharmaceutical analyses, the measurement methods used by mass spectrometry include selected − ion monitoring (SIM), selective reaction monitoring (SRM), or multi reaction monitoring (MRM). the external or internal standard method is used for quantitation. When using the standard curve method, the response of series of standard solutions are recorded. A calibration curve is created by reference standards responses versus their concentrations. Prepare the test solution as described in the monograph, record the characteristic response of ions (m/z). The concentration of component is calculated by the calibration curve.

3. Apparatus and Reagents

3.1 Apparatus

High performance liquid chromatograph system; Triple quadrupole mass spectrometry; Analytical balance; Centrifuge; Ultrasonic cleaning instrument; Volumetric flask (50ml, 10ml); Flask (100ml); Transfer pipette (1ml).

3.2 Reagents

Toosendan Fructus, Toosendanin reference substance (purity is more than 99%); Acetonitrile, methanol and formic acid are HPLC grade reagent; Nitrogen and argon (purity is more than 99.999%); Water is deionized.

4. Experimental contents

4.1 Preparation of the reference solution

Accurately weigh toosendanin reference substance to a 10ml volumetric flask, then dissolve and dilute with methanol solution to prepare the stock solution of toosendanin (100μg/ml). Take 1ml of the stock solution to a 50ml volumetric flask, then further diluted with methanol solution to obtain the reference solution (2μg/ml).

4. 2 Preparation of the test solution

Place 0.25g of the powdered material (through No.4 sieve), accurately weighed, in a 100ml round bottom flask. Accurately add 50ml of methanol and weigh, heating circumfluence for 1hour, then cool to room temperature and weigh, readjust to the original weight with methanol. Shake and filter through a microporous membrane (0.22μm) to obtain the test solution.

4. 3 Chromatographic conditions

Hypersil GOLD C_{18} (50mm × 2.1mm, 3μm) or similar columns is used as the stationary phase. Water (containing 0.01% formic acid) – acetonitrile (69 : 31) are used as the mobile phase with the flow rate of 0.2ml/min and column temperature of 35℃. The injection volume is set to 2.0μl.

4. 4 LC – MS conditions

All analyses are carried out in negative – ion or positive – ion ESI mode with multiple reaction monitoring (MRM). Sheath gas is nitrogen and collision gasis argon. Other operating parameters, such as collision energy, spray voltage, and ionization temperature, are automatically optimized by the instrument. The chromatographic retention time and characteristic fragments of toosendanin standard are used for qualitative and quantitative analysis.

4. 5 Condition optimization

Toosendanin standard is scanned on the range of m/z 100 – 800 in negative – ion or positive – ion ESI mode, the most appropriate electrospray ionization mode and molecular ion peak are selected for analysis. Based on the precursor ion and MS/MS product ions by secondary mass scanning, the most abundant fragment ions with less interference are used as qualitative and quantitative ions. The monitoring ions m/z 573.3→425.3 and m/z 573.3→531.4 are selected for reference. The MS/MS conditions are optimized for the optimum sensitivity.

4. 6 Calibration curve

The stock solution of toosendanin (100μg/ml) is further diluted with mobile phase to obtain standard solutions of 0.05μg/ml, 0.25μg/ml, 0.50μg/ml, 1.00μg/ml, 5.00μg/ml, 10.00 μg/ml and 50.00μg/ml. There are two tautomers of toosendanin because of the hemiacetal structure. Thus the calibration curve is constructed by plotting the sum of peak areas of two tautomers (Y) versus the concentration (X) using weighted linear least square regression.

4. 7 Limit of detection (LOD) and limit of quantitation (LOQ)

The stock solution oftoosendanin is serially diluted with mobile phase, and the peak areas at the retention time are recorded. The limit of detection (LOD) and limit of quantification (LOQ) are defined as the amounts of the analytes at a signal – to – noise ratio (S/N) of 3.0 and 10.0, respectively.

4. 8 Precision

Take one batch of the Toosendan Fructus materials, process them as directed under the "Preparation of the test solution" to obtain the test solution, then consecutive inject for six times. The precision is defined as the relative standard deviation (RSD) of the toosendanin peak areas.

4.9 Repeatability

Take one batch of theToosendan Fructus materials, process them as directed under the "Preparation of the test solution" to obtain six test solutions. After analysis, the contents of toosendanin are determined. The repeatability is defined as the RSD of the contents of six test solutions.

4.10 Stability

Take one batch of theToosendan Fructus materials, process them as directed under the "Preparation of the test solution" to obtain the test solution, then inject the sample under 0h, 1h, 2h, 4h, 8h, 12h and 24h. The peak areas of toosendanin are recorded. The stability is defined as the RSD of toosendanin peak areas under different times.

4.11 Recovery

Accurately weigh nine samples of 0.12g Toosendan Fructus materials (known content), add toosendanin standard at low, medium and high (80μg, 160μg and 240μg) levels of 3 replicates, process them according to the "Preparation of the test solution". The recovery is determined by comparing the contents of toosendanin detected that added in samples with the corresponding standards.

4.12 Contents (μg/g) of toosendanin in samples

Accurately weigh Toosendan Fructus materials, process them as directed under the "Preparation of the test solution" to obtain the test solutions. Each sample is injected into LC – MS system for 3 times and the peak areas are recorded. The concentration of toosendanin are calculated according to calibration curve.

5. Data record and processing

5.1 Precursor ion and product ions

Table 19 – 1　The electrospray ionization mode

Mode	Precursor ion (m/z)	Product ions (m/z)
positive – ion mode		
negative – ion mode		

5.2 Results of calibration curve, LOD and LOQ

Table 19 – 2　Results of calibration curve

No.	Retention time (min)	Concentration (μg/ml)	Peak area
1			
2			
3			
4			
5			
6			
7			

Regression equation		Correlation coefficient (r)	
LOD		LOQ	

5.3 Results of precision

Table 19－3　Results of precision

No.	Retention time (min)	Peak area	Mean peak area	RSD(%)
1				
2				
3				
4				
5				
6				

5.4 Results of repeatability

Table 19－4　Results of repeatability

No.	Amount (g)	Peak area	Content (μg/g)	Mean content (μg/g)	RSD(%)
1					
2					
3					
4					
5					
6					

5.5 Results of stability

Table 19－5　Results of stability

Storage time (h)	Retention time (min)	Peak area	RSD(%)
0			
1			
2			
4			
8			
12			
24			

5.6 Results ofrecovery

Table 19－6　Results of recovery

No.	Original (μg)	Spiked (μg)	Found (μg)	Recovery (%)	Mean recovery (%)	RSD (%)
1		80				
2		80				
3		80				
4		160				
5		160				
6		160				
7		240				
8		240				
9		240				

5. 7 Results oftoosendanin contents (μg/g)in samples

Table 19 – 7　Results of toosendanin contents (μg/g)in samples

No.	Batch	Amount(g)	Peak area	Content (μg/g)	Mean content (μg/g)
1					
2					
3					
4					
5					
6					

6. Discussion and guidance

6. 1 Precautions of LC – MS mobile phase

Mobile phase and samples should filter through a microporous membrane(0. 22μm)before injection. Ultrasonic degassing of mobile phase (or online degassing device)is for the stability of the pressure. Make sure there is enough solvent in the reservoir and never run the column dry. LC – MS mobile phase often consisted of methanol, acetonitrile, water and volatile buffer, for example, ammonium formate, ammonium acetate, formic acid and acetic acid etc. The involatile salts, such as phosphate, citrate etc and ion – pair reagent do not match LC – MS system, because high concentration of involatile salts would decrease ionization effect, block spray needle and contaminate instruments.

6. 2 The optimization of mass conditions

The appropriate electrospray ionization mode depends on the structural information of the analyte. When the determined components are basic compounds such as secondary amine or tertiary amine (sulfonamides or quinolones etc), formic acid or acetic acid are always added to acidulate mobile phase. When the determined components are acid compounds with negative groups such as chlorinum, bromine or hydroxyl (chloramphenicol etc), ammonia is always added to mobile phase for basification.

6. 3 Methods used for measurement

The following methods are used for measurements using mass spectrometry. An outline of the data obtained by each method is also described.

a. Full scan mode　Full scan mode is also known as the total ion monitoring (TIM). It is the technique in which the mass spectrometer is operated so that all ions within the selected *m/z* range are detected and recorded, and the integrated value of the amounts of ions observed in each scanning is called the total ion current (TIC).

The chromatogram in which the total ion current obtained from the mass spectrummeasured in LC – MS is plotted against the retention time is called the total ion current chromatogram (TICC), and the chromatogram in which the relative intensity at the specific *m/z* value is expressed as the function of time is called the extracted ion chromatogram (EIC).

b. Selected ion monitoring (SIM)　In selected ion monitoring (SIM), the mass spectrometer is operated so that only the ions with a specific m/z value are continuously detected and recorded instead of measuring the mass spectrum. SIM is used for the assay and high – sensitivity detection of sample substances in LC – MS.

c. Product – ionscan   The precursor ions are obtained from first mass analyzer, then production scan is used to scan the product ions that generated from the precursor ions with the selected m/z range from second mass analyzer. With this method, the mass spectrum of precursor ions can be obtained.

d. Precursor – ion scan   Precursor ion scan is a method for scanning the precursor ions from which the product ions with a specific m/z value are generated by dissociation, and it is used for the specific detection of a substance with a specified substructure in the sample.

e. Neutral – loss scan   In neutral – loss scan, the precursor ions that undergo the loss of specified mass (desorption of neutral species) due to dissociation are scanned. This method is used for the specific detection of substances with a specified neutral fragment (e. g. CO_2) in the sample.

f. Selected reaction monitoring (SRM)   Selected reaction monitoring (SRM) detects product ions with a specific m/z value generated by the dissociation of the precursor ions with a specified m/z value, and it is used for the quantitative detection of trace amounts of substances present in a complex matrix. Although this method is similar to SIM, the specificity is improved by using the product ions generated from the precursor ions for the detection.

6. 4 Validation of analysis method

The purpose ofvalidation of analysis method is to ensure that the adopted method meets the requirements for the intended analytical applications. The analytical items that must be verified include identification, quantification or limit test of impurities, content determination of the active ingredients in drug substance or preparation and that of other components in the preparation, such as antiseptic, other residue in herb medicine, and additives etc. The parameters of validation characteristics include accuracy, precision (including repeatability, intermediate – precision and reproducibility), specificity, limit of detection, limit of quantitation, linearity, range and ruggedness. The validation of analysis method is determined with standard substance.

扫码"练一练"